Individuality and Ideology in British Object Relations Theory

"What could be timelier than a book that illuminates the path from maternal holding and caretaking to active citizenship, peaceful civilizations, and the promotion of redistributive social policies?"

Michael A. Diamond, *Professor Emeritus of Public Affairs and Organization Studies, University of Missouri*

"Gerson usefully illuminates the often obscured ethico-political vision underpinning competing schools of psychodynamic thought and practice—specifically, their underlying patriarchal or matriarchal orientation."

Don Carveth, *Emeritus Professor of Sociology and Social & Political Thought, Senior Scholar, York University*

Following the work of prominent object relations theorists, such as Fairbairn, Suttie and Winnicott, Gal Gerson explores the correlation between analytical theory and intellectual environment in two ways. He notes the impact that the British object relations school had on both psychology and wider culture, and suggests that the school's outlook involved more than a clinical choice.

Gerson first interprets the object relations model as a political theory that completes a certain internal development within liberalism. He later outlines the relationship between the analytical theory and the historical setting in which it formed and took root. By engaging with these questions, Gerson demonstrates the deeper structure and implications of object relation theory for social philosophy. This allows him to answer questions such as: 'What kind of social arrangements do we endorse when we accept object relations theory as a fair description of mind?'; 'What beliefs about power, individuality, and household structure do we take in? What do we give up when doing so?'; and, lastly, 'What does it say about contemporary advanced societies that they have taken in much of the theory's content?'

Proposing a novel rethinking of human nature, *Individuality and Ideology in British Object Relations Theory* provides much-needed insight into how this school of psychoanalytic theory has impacted contemporary social and political life.

Gal Gerson *teaches political theory and the history of political thought at the University of Haifa, Israel*

Psychoanalytic Political Theory

Edited by Matthew H. Bowker, Medaille College and David W. McIvor, Colorado State University

Psychoanalytic Political Theory provides a publishing space for the highest quality scholarship at the intersection of psychoanalysis and normative political theory. It offers a forum for texts that deepen our understanding of the complex relationships between the world of politics and the world of the psyche.

Recently Published Books

1 **The Lucid Vigil**
Deconstruction, Desire and the Politics of Critique
Stella Gaon

2 **Individuality and Ideology in British Object Relations Theory**
Gal Gerson

Individuality and Ideology in British Object Relations Theory

Gal Gerson

Routledge
Taylor & Francis Group
NEW YORK AND LONDON

First published 2021
by Routledge
52 Vanderbilt Avenue, New York, NY 10017

and by Routledge
2 Park Square, Milton Park, Abingdon, Oxon, OX14 4RN

Routledge is an imprint of the Taylor & Francis Group, an informa business

Library of Congress Cataloging-in-Publication Data
Names: Gerson, Gal, 1964– author.
Title: Individuality and ideology in British object relations theory : from the cradle and on / Gal Gerson.
Description: New York, NY : Routledge, 2021. |
Series: Psychoanalytic political theory ; vol 2 |
Includes bibliographical references and index.
Identifiers: LCCN 2020058238 (print) |
LCCN 2020058239 (ebook) | ISBN 9781138333154 (hardback) |
ISBN 9780429446146 (ebook) | ISBN 9780429820823 (adobe pdf) |
ISBN 9780429820809 (mobi) | ISBN 9780429820816 (epub)
Subjects: LCSH: Object relations (Psychoanalysis)—
Great Britain. | Individuality—Great Britain.
Classification: LCC BF175.5.O24 G37 2021 (print) |
LCC BF175.5.O24 (ebook) | DDC 150.19/5—dc23
LC record available at https://lccn.loc.gov/2020058238
LC ebook record available at https://lccn.loc.gov/2020058239

ISBN: 978-1-138-33315-4 (hbk)
ISBN: 978-0-367-76165-3 (pbk)
ISBN: 978-0-429-44614-6 (ebk)

Typeset in Times New Roman
by codeMantra

Contents

Introduction

Object relations psychoanalysis can justly claim credit for its influence on society and culture. Emanating from modifications of Freud's theory, the idea that the mind is structured around internalized images of very early parental inputs has become prevalent in therapeutic thinking and practice. The legacy of the object relations approach has fused with the popular image of psychotherapy and psychology themselves (Clarke, 2006: 9). While psychoanalysis is still identified with the classical terminology of the oedipal situation and erotogenic zones, the second half of the twentieth century has become equally acquainted with notions taken from the object relations literature, such as maternal deprivation, transitional objects and the goodenough mother. Ideas based on object relations theory inform disciplines that are adjacent to psychology, such as social work, education, sociology and criminology. Through the multiplication of therapeutic, counselling and coaching practices, ideas rooted in object relations theory have migrated into the terms and languages of everyday experience in ways far removed from the original, midcentury context in which these notions had been formulated. This broad impact points at the ability of that particular psychoanalytical school to reflect, respond to, and possibly modulate, the sensibilities of its time.

Scholarship has been slow to take note of these many connections between object relations theory and the surrounding society. While Freudian theory has caught the attention of historical, philosophical and sociological research, object relations theory's makeup and implications are more seldom considered in such terms. Possibly, this relative neglect emanates from the same factors that allowed the contents of object relations theory to be so prevalently disseminated. Object relations analysts were not intentionally social iconoclasts. Without the sense of outrage that attended Freud's reception, engagement with their theory remained localized within the orbit of their own and neighbouring professions, drawing limited attention from social or political scholars. But this continuity itself makes the content of object relations theory worthy of additional consideration. It entails that the analysts added detail and coherence to an already existing ideology and thus triggered no overt counter-reaction. Their works can be read as texts in the history of political thought.

Nonetheless, some researches on the social historical and political implications of object relations have been conducted. They point to the theory's connections with the formation of the welfare state in Britain. The term refers here to the aggregate of governmental service-delivering bodies along with the legislation, administrative policies and economic measures meant to facilitate the operation of these bodies, as these emerged in Britain and in other Western countries during the 1930s and 1940s.

Researchers have noted two kinds of such links between object relations theory and the ideology of the liberal welfare state. The first is sociological and organizational. Forged during a time of war and mass displacement, object relations theory focuses on the concerns of a society grappling with crisis. As it emphasizes the crucial role of the family environment, object relations thought correspondingly stresses the adverse results of separation and loss. The theory therefore entails guidelines for action calibrated to minimize such harm to individuals and families while stabilizing and preserving valued social practices (Homans, 1989: 227–229; Riley, 1983; van der Horst and van der Veer, 2010). Clinicians' ideas about the roles of motherhood, the family household and education frequently served as material for public policies, as embedded, for example, in the Children Act of 1948 (Jones, 1960: 147–152). Implementing these policies was the responsibility of the welfare apparatus as it developed in the 1930s and 1940s. Psychologists worked alongside and within the public agencies charged with health and education. Their thinking was enmeshed with the practices, ideas and prejudices that characterized these organizations, as pointed out by Butler (2020), Mayhew (2006), Rose (1985, 1996) and Shapira (2013).

The second type of connection between object relations theory and the welfare state is more focused on the intellectual and philosophical contents of the ideas that the psychoanalytical theory upholds. Object relations psychoanalysis regards individuality, personal freedom and creativity as conditioned on the individual's early environment, and therefore as essentially social: the analysts understand the formation of the coherent, benevolent and autonomously acting personality as predicated on the availability of a nourishing setting and attentive parent. With varying emphases, Alexander (2012), Etheridge (1977), Gerson (2004), Groarke (2014), Hoggett (2008), Rustin (1991) and Zaretsky (2004: 249–275) point out that believing in such a relationship between social provision and individual agency concurs with the advanced liberal and social-democratic thinking that underlined the construction of the redistributive, welfare-oriented polity. Within the broad contours of this ideology, personal freedom is the cherished end, while environmental support is the indispensable means. By providing an account of how the link between support and autonomy works on the level of the individual person's mind, object relations theory accords with the ideas that shored up the welfare-state agenda associated with William Beveridge's 1942 Plan.

Welfare-state thought displays another trait beside its wish to guarantee sufficient social conditions for the development of a free, self-determining individuality. The intellectual input that went into the making of the welfare state favoured the expansion of governmental provision, but, true to its roots in historical liberal philosophy, not of state authority. The welfare state was forged to address an essential and integrative, not technical, perception of society's needs. Planning, redistribution and the expansion of services were tied to a set of concepts that pertained to human life in its holistic entirety. The formulation 'from the cradle to the grave' that attached to it captures this feature: welfare-state thought aspired to neglect no corner of our experience (Fraser, 2017: 14). As the state could not simply be trusted with powers over such an expanse of issues, advanced liberals sought to render the state and its government secondary to a federative alignment of everyday contacts and forms of cooperation, voluntary associations, and wider, regional and global governance systems. This advanced liberalism assumed that individuals who enjoy the social safety network furnished by their polity would form into a self-regulating civilization in which the coercive, force-wielding function of government would diminish. Politics in the conventional sense would become a more marginal issue than before.

Here, I argue that, when examined as a political theory, object relations thought matches this character of the advanced liberal approach developed in the first half of the twentieth century. To different degrees and with considerable variations, the psychoanalysts think of the civic politics that takes place around sovereign institutions as at best a regrettable necessity, expecting its significance to decline if the conditions for a healthy democracy are maintained. The expectation of a diminished politics was essential enough for it to be retained within object relations thought even once the setting has changed from its midcentury configuration. In later elaborations of the theory, the vision of a benign, natural social mode that gradually obviates existential disagreement and the organs mandated to channel it is upheld and occasionally made more explicit.

The Argument: Outline and Section Sequence

As the current scholarly consensus establishes, object relations theory formed within the intellectual climate that made possible the justification of a more interventionist state from liberal and individualist premises. In early-twentieth century and midcentury Britain, that justification included the perception of sociability as a constitutive human character that generates a universal right to engage with other individuals in multiple sites and locations. Emphasizing this trait made it feasible for liberal and individualist thinkers to task government with offering channels for sociability to unfold. Liberal reformers valued sociability for several reasons, among which the period's circumstances played a crucial role. On the one hand, industrial society caused alienation and seemed to encourage a turn towards illiberal ideologies that promised a more communal existence. On the other hand, the same industrial conditions offered venues for communication and, consequently, for personal development, an end compatible with the values of constitutional democracy itself as understood by these thinkers. To compete with its illiberal detractors while making good use of the new conditions, liberalism rephrased itself in terms that highlighted the function of interpersonal closeness. Reforming liberals played up the concept of the human individual as other-seeking, using that concept as a lynchpin that connected the differing historical perceptions of individual liberty. Government was charged with preserving the conditions where natural society's bodies could thrive but also with protecting each person's autonomy and ability to associate within these bodies. While expanding the state's responsibilities, this concept did not extend the state's authority to the same extent. Freely and spontaneously engaging with each other, democratic subjects were creative: together, they produced ideas and goods that they could not have alone. One of the things they created together was new forums for engagement. Hence, while natural in the sense of preceding the state, the society made of these multiple engagements was not fixed in scope. Its practices and mental habits could develop to the degree of permeating the sphere of government. Politics could cease to be a region for the work of power and conflicting interests. Fears of bureaucratic invasion into privacy could be allayed, as governmental offices were the arms of a multilayered and complex civilization based on mutually interested individuals. Reforming liberals presented the expanded apparatus required by the welfare state as assisting the region of liberty, privacy, dynamic creativity and personal contacts rather than as an imposition on that region.

The vision of a private sphere which, when acknowledged and protected by political institutions, curbs the conflictual dimension of politics appeared in more ideologies than welfare-oriented liberalism. The realization that the world's different parts were irrevocably linked and that war could not be kept local meant that many who did not necessarily agree with the welfare agenda shared its concern with allowing a space for freely created ties to unfold so as to tame the expressly political, force-wielding bodies. The ideal of a worldwide, plural system that empowers the multiple overlapping and dynamic interactions entered voluntarily by individuals was gaining traction. It was shared, with varying emphases, by ideological positions on the left and right of welfare-state liberalism. It was provided with a comprehensive philosophical argument – as well as a popular catchphrase – by Popper's notion of the open society. These right, left and centre ideologies shaped public and scholarly debates about the postwar world. The growing trust in, and corresponding willingness to calibrate government to cultivate, the various activities, associations and groupings individuals are believed to wish to enter and generate on their own can be seen as a kind of zeitgeist, a rising agreement on what freedom and democracy were.

Object relations theory matched these outlooks by offering a view of the individual mind that was similarly organized around a sociable motivation whose manifestations could branch out gradually until they enfolded the forums tasked with collective decision and enforcement. Initiating the creation of object relations theory as an independent and distinctly British approach in a series of observations since the 1920s, Ian Suttie and Jane Suttie located a tender, other-seeking motivation at the core of psychic development, replacing Freud's sexualized notion of libido and allowing for the construction of the mother-dominated family as the site where any tendency towards violence is pre-empted. In the 1930s, Ronald Fairbairn anchored a comparable belief in a governing sociable motivation to the structured and tidily argued terms of a psychoanalytic model. Fairbairn reinterpreted Melanie Klein's view of destructive instincts and the part-objects they create as reflecting the work of an integrative and sociable drive. Fairbairn described these drives and objects as a matrix generated by the interaction of different other-seeking strategies the very young child engages in. Starting later in that decade, Donald Winnicott further elaborated these insights by formulating the concept of a transitional space for play and creativity opened up between child and parent. Pervaded by its search for validation, the self becomes able to tolerate, and then value, difference and disagreement, thus constantly proceeding towards a more integrated, confident and explorative existence. Tensions and frictions are foils for the wish to engage with others, and assist its growing sophistication. As confidence, exploration and movement are themselves conditioned by the experience of early attachment, autonomy means that healthy individuals create further attachments through new friendships, families, collegial affiliations, professional achievements and other activities that derive their significance from the experience they offer individuals of being witnessed and responded to by others. Together, these activities constitute an intermediate world accessible to all and incrementally impacted by all. For the Sutties, Fairbairn and Winnicott alike, society as a whole was tasked with providing conditions in which the secure household could function. As its function was creative and dynamic, the products of this protected private sphere could be expected to enfold the entire society, including its political and civic spaces. In Winnicott's particular formulation, these ideas are compatible with the notions of the democratic civilization as described at the time by Popper.

Decades later, far from the midcentury British setting in which the Sutties, Fairbairn and Winnicott worked, Jessica Benjamin developed a comprehensive, expressly political and social theory from object relations premises. It replicates and accentuates some of the features that appeared in more implicit ways in the midcentury analysts. Like the Sutties, Benjamin views the empowerment of mothers and women as the key to individual and social health. With Winnicott, she stresses the self-healing and dynamically creative character of differences when tested, asserted and survived in a validating environment. The resulting outlook is expressly critical of the Hobbesian perception according to which lethal violence and the organs tasked with it are central to human existence. Such perceptions, Benjamin maintains, normalize the pathology of a self that is preoccupied with power dualities, hierarchic distinctions, boundaries and classifications. The overall trend towards expanding the patterns based on the domestic, intimate and emotional private sphere to the point where the politics of public, impersonal and force-wielding institutions become secondary and possibly redundant is explicitly central in Benjamin, placing into relief an ideological feature that existed in object relations theory all along.

This is the mainstay of the argument here. It is presented in six chapters. The first is a general description of the ideas about the distinction of politics and its relationship with the private existence of individuals and households, as they appeared in both the reforming liberalism of the early to mid-twentieth-century welfare state and in the object relations literature. The second and third chapters discuss two early versions of the ideological notions involved in object relations psychoanalysis: the more optimistic, borderline-utopian vision offered by Ian Suttie and Jane Suttie, and the comparatively dour and lowkey version laid out by Ronald Fairbairn. The fourth chapter is devoted to Donald Winnicott's ideas about the link between the home, healthy or otherwise, the experiences and social venues based on the home, and the political realm. It is followed by a comparison of Winnicott's views with those of Popper in the fifth chapter, and then by an account of Benjamin's contribution in the sixth chapter.

Boundaries and Disclaimers

This essay relies on existing research, whose descriptions and assertions it basically takes for granted as its axiomatic basis. It relies on the historiography that depicts the development of Anglophone, mainly British, liberal thought from a minimalist creed that sought to shelter individuals' private lives into a more interventionist platform, in which governmental acts, planning and day-to-day involvement are beneficent for personal freedom. The classical liberal positions that served as the basis of this transformation are generally those of John Locke and J.S. Mill, and to a differing degree, those of Edmund Burke and Lord Acton. Their revision was carried out in the twentieth century by scholars, journalists and policy planners, like Leonard Hobhouse; John Hobson; and, later, William

Beveridge and T.H. Marshall (Backhouse, Bateman, and Nishizawa, 2017; Clarke, 1978; Freeden, 1978; Jackson, 2007). This essay depends, additionally, on the research literature that traces the controversy within political thought between the individualist liberalism that focused on the single person as the carrier of rights, and the more pluralist approach that stressed the role of voluntary associations as defences against governmental power. One occurrence within this development was the endorsement of pluralist elements into the way democracy was understood since the 1940s in the Atlantic West (Levy, 2015; Rosenboim, 2017). I take my view of object relations theory's origins, development, content and boundaries from accounts that name Ian Suttie, Ronald Fairbairn, John Bowlby and Donald Winnicott as some of its main authors, and describe these authors' differences from Freud and Klein as serious enough to identify them as a distinct and roughly cohesive psychoanalytic school (Gomez, 1997; Greenberg and Mitchell, 1983; Rayner, 1990; Schwartz, 1999; Symington, 2014).

Based on these accounts of the welfare state's grounding in liberal philosophy, the pluralist influx into consensual views of democracy and the formation of object relations theory, this essay attempts to connect them. It does so by discussing how the contents of object relations theory match the view of politics entailed by a certain range of mainly liberal political and social authors. Accordingly, this essay is primarily a text on the history of political thought, in which the sources happen to be composed of psychoanalytical literature. It treats that literature as a private case of a wider transformation within social thought, and details some of the causes and effects of this transformation where such details are relevant to object relations thought. It stakes no claims on the clinical, medical or therapeutic validity of object relations psychoanalysis or any other method of treatment.

I wish to thank the team at Routledge, in particular the series editors, Matt Bowker and David McIvor, for their helpful suggestions and supportive attitude. The organizers and participants of Graham Clarke's and David Scharff's 2014 symposium on Fairbairn at the Freud Museum, London, gave a favourable and fruitful welcome to some of the ideas printed here. I have been fortunate in having an uncommonly tolerant and cooperative work environment at the University of Haifa, enabled and daily maintained throughout the challenges of institutional life by my divisional colleagues Ayelet Banai, Daphna Canetti, As'ad Ghanem, Liran Harsgor, Annabel Herzog, Doron Navot, Aviad Rubin, and Israel Waismel-Manor.

Parts of Chapter 2 in this essay are reproduced with the permission of the American Psychological Association from an article that was originally published as:

Gerson, G. (2009). Culture and ideology in Ian Suttie's theory of mind. *History of Psychology* 12 (1): 19–40.

Elements of Chapter 3 in this essay are reproduced with permission from Taylor and Francis through PLSclear from a chapter contribution that originally appeared as:

Gerson, G. (2014). From Oedipus to Antigone: Hegelian themes in Fairbairn. In Scharff, D., and Clarke, G.S. (eds.), *Fairbairn and the object relations tradition*. London: Karnac, 27–39.

Elements of Chapter 4 in this essay are reproduced with the permission included in the guidelines announced by Sage from articles that originally appeared as the following two articles:

Gerson, G. (2004). Winnicott, participation and gender. *Feminism & Psychology* 14 (4): 561–581.

Gerson, G. (2005). Individuality, deliberation and welfare in Donald Winnicott. *History of the Human Sciences* 18 (1): 107–126.

References

Alexander, S. (2012). Primary maternal preoccupation: D.W. Winnicott and social democracy in mid-twentieth-century Britain. In Alexander, S., and Taylor, B. (eds.), *History and psyche: Culture, psychoanalysis, and the past*. New York: Palgrave, 149–172.

Backhouse, R.E., Bateman B.W., and Nishizawa, T. (2017). Liberalism and the welfare state in Britain, 1890–1945. In Backhouse, R.E., Bateman B.W., Nishizawa, T., and Plehwe, D. (eds.), *Liberalism and the welfare state*. Oxford: Oxford University Press, 25–38.

Butler, L. (2020). *Michael Young, social science and the British left 1945–1970*. Oxford: Oxford University Press.

Clarke, G.S. (2006). *Personal relations theory*. London: Routledge.

Clarke, P.F. (1978). *Liberals and social democrats*. Cambridge: Cambridge University Press.

Etheridge, L. (1977). Optimal federalism: A model of psychological dependence. *Policy Sciences* 8: 161–171.

Fraser, D. (2017). *The evolution of the British welfare state*. Fifth edition. London: Palgrave.

Freeden, M.S. (1978). *The new liberalism*. Oxford: Clarendon.

Gerson, G. (2004). Object relations psychoanalysis as political theory. *Political Psychology* 25 (5): 769–794.

Gomez, L. (1997). *An introduction to object relations*. New York: New York University Press.

Greenberg, J.R., and Mitchell, S.A. (1983). *Object relations in psychoanalytic theory*. Cambridge, MA and London: Harvard University Press.

Groarke, S. (2014). *Managed lives*. London: Routledge.

Hoggett, P. (2008). Relational thinking and welfare practice. In Clarke, S., Hahn, H., and Hoggett, P. (eds.), *Object relations and social relations*. London: Karnac, 65–86.

Homans, P. (1989). *The ability to mourn*. Chicago, IL and London: The University of Chicago Press.

Horst, F.C.P van der, and Veer, R. van der. (2010). The ontogeny of an idea: John Bowlby and contemporaries on mother-child separation. *History of Psychology* 13 (1): 25–45.

Jackson, B. (2007). *Equality and the British left.* Manchester: Manchester University Press.
Jones, K. (1960). *Mental health and social policy.* London: Routledge & Kegan Paul.
Levy, J.T. (2015). *Rationalism, pluralism, and freedom.* Oxford: Oxford University Press.
Mayhew, B. (2006). Between love and aggression: The politics of John Bowlby. *History of the Human Sciences* 19 (4): 19–35.
Rayner, E. (1990). *The independent mind in British psychoanalysis.* London: Free Association.
Riley, D. (1983). *War in the nursery.* London: Virago.
Rose, N. (1985) *The psychological complex.* London: Routledge & Kegan Paul.
Rose, N. (1996). *Inventing our selves.* Cambridge: Cambridge University Press.
Rosenboim, O. (2017). *The emergence of globalism.* Princeton, NJ: Princeton University Press.
Rustin, M. (1991). *The good society and the inner world.* London and New York: Verso.
Schwartz, J. (1999). *Cassandra's daughter.* London: Penguin.
Shapira, M. (2013). *The war inside.* Cambridge: Cambridge University Press.
Symington, N. (2014). Fairbairn, Suttie and Macmurray – An essay. In Clarke, G.S., and Scharff, D.E., *Fairbairn and the object relations tradition.* London: Karnac, 59–67.
Zaretsky, E. (2004). *Secrets of the soul: A social and cultural history of psychoanalysis.* New York: Alfred Knopf.

1 Individual Interiors and the Liberal Order

The revision of Freudian theory into object relations psychoanalysis took place while the society where object relations theorists lived was beginning to translate a certain development within political theory into concrete policies and public bodies. Ideas which have been brewing among intellectuals and journalists since the beginning of the twentieth century morphed during the 1940s into the agenda, and then the institutions, of the welfare state. This development was at once a response to the everyday, practical problems of a society mired in economic crisis, uncertainty and war, and an attempt to streamline the older body of liberal concepts into a practicable creed that matched the time's realities. Object relations theory meshed into this development by providing the liberal welfare agenda with a view of the mind that was informed by a structured model and enjoyed the prestige of a discipline that was considered innovative for its time. Object relations psychoanalysis also displays some consistent parallels with the revised liberal philosophy on which the welfare state was based.

In the immediately following section of this chapter I offer a broad-lensed view of the time. Marred by war and dislocation, the twentieth century's first half was considered alternatively as a catastrophic time for democracy itself, for the enlightened civilization on which it was based and for liberal thinking, and as an opportunity for the development and growth of enlightenment, liberalism and democracy. In Britain, where liberal tenets were woven into the national history and collective image, the contradicting stakes for political theory were placed into a sharper relief, leading to a thorough revision of liberal ideas and to their synthesis into a new, welfare-oriented agenda. This process is described in the second section of this chapter as an internal debate within liberal philosophy. A short, third part examines some of the broader cultural meanings of this development. Returning to the discussion of psychoanalytical thought, the succeeding three parts examine the parallels between object relations theory and the advanced liberalism of its time in three thematic fields: the crucial role of sociability, the belief in the creative and expansive character of the society that acknowledges sociability, and the policy recommendations that follow from these ideas.

The Crisis and Resurgence of Liberalism

Since its inception in the last decade of the nineteenth century, psychoanalysis featured as both a threat and an ally to the constitutional, democratic and liberal view of politics. The more negative view places psychoanalysis within an overall decline of the rational, individualist and progress-oriented approach to social affairs. The twentieth century could no longer believe in the combination of free market, individualism and scientific rationalism. Capitalism generated inequality and poverty. Expanding communications exposed profound incompatibilities in outlook and values within each society, while highlighting the difficulty of fruitful dialogue between societies. Scientific knowledge accumulated only to gnaw at its own basis. Darwinian biology replaced the ordered tree of the species by a trajectory of arbitrary extinctions. Social-science research suggested that civilization is conditioned by the contagion of crowds and the embedded power of elites rather than shaped by respectful conversation among responsible citizens. And Freud's psychology showed that each apparently rational adult is a compendium of archaic, actively forgotten and nameless wishes and fears. The upshot of these revelations was mutually reflected by politics in the form of nationalist and revolutionary movements that placed collective before individual and turned to violence as a legitimate means. The eruption of the world wars and the rise of totalitarianism further manifested the implications of the broader, cultural and intellectual undercurrents. A deadlocked world shot through with the fear of nuclear extinction followed these wars. Instead of constitutional societies made of distinct and enlightened individuals and ruled by universally respected laws, one was looking at gigantic ant heaps governed by crushing hierarchies and liable to ferociously throw themselves at each other on the first suitable occasion. Liberal thinkers in this atmosphere became dour and pessimistic (Bellamy, 2003; Eksteins, 1990; Fawcett, 2014: 286–289, 332–338; Gerson, 2004: 13–18; Herman, 1997: 109–145; Kern, 1983).

But, by ordering the data differently, a more upbeat narrative about the twentieth century's first half becomes possible. Rather than being cowed by the apparent advent of irrationality, mass culture and conflictual politics, liberalism utilized them to create a broader and more complex perception of liberty. Freedom, it was now realized, had to be shielded not only from the arbitrary power of government, but also from the dangers newly exposed by science and history: rampant capitalism, mass suggestion, the subtle hold of social and cultural mediators, and the power dynamics that unfold even in the most intimate social units. A broadened perception of liberty as the right to be respected, educated, healed and heard by others was established as a guideline for Western societies. It extended to the international arena, where its tenets were endorsed as the basis of the ideal world order declared by the

Atlantic Charter. Liberalism's expansion was accompanied by developments in knowledge that everywhere, from physics to philosophy, emphasized complexity, multiplicity and relativity. The strict certainties that in the Victorian mind had linked appearance to essence and so validated wealth as a manifestation of virtue were substituted by a more tolerant perspective. Diversity in experience and outlook was increasingly welcomed as highlighting broader aspects of a shared world and grounding a more generous and inclusive notion of individual rights (Fawcett, 2014: 286–302). In this more optimistic account of liberalism's fate, psychoanalysis plays the role of catalyzing the recognition that the human persona is wider than its visible and socially accepted parts. Psychoanalysis showed that individual autonomy needed active fostering and therapeutic attention. The ego was to be empowered, not by denying id, but by acknowledging it. Desire and creativity were as necessary for a sense of individual agency as were instrumental reason and the acquisition of skills (Roazen, 2003; West, 1986).

The contrast between the two narratives stands out particularly in the discussion of British history. A tested constitutional polity marked by a traditional respect for law that obviated the armed police and gendarmerie characteristic of other European countries, early twentieth-century Britain was at the same time burdened by archaic practices that tainted its commitment to liberty. Its society was riven by inequalities that seared themselves into the national image. Pessimist histories of British liberalism stress the high, even terminal price paid by liberalism for indulging these contradictions. Their consequences made it to the surface in the first decade of the century, when imperialism and the divided loyalties of Ireland asserted themselves in strident, extraparliamentary forms of activism. The First World War saw Britain issuing a conscription order that countered its homegrown dislike of a standing army. Soon, that army was deployed to quell Britain's rebelling Irish citizens (Dangerfield, 1935). With the last Liberal-Party administration leaving office in 1922, British political life was taken over by conservatism and socialism. With the mediating, constitutionalist position compromised, direct action and force seemed to prevail. By the 1930s, nationwide strikes, demonstrations and marches overshadowed the politics of voting and representation. Ideologies previously dismissed as unrealistically purist and extreme, such as pacifism and fascism, were given unprecedented scope. Optimist accounts of British liberalism, by contrast, emphasize that the same decades witnessed the enfranchisement of women, the scaling-down of capital punishment, the replacement of the punitive and antiquated Poor Laws by a more systemic attention to social needs, and the streamlining of the country's laws and practices along more egalitarian principles. The fundamentals of parliamentary representation and civil rights were preserved, alongside the respect for personal discretion in private life, throughout the tumult of war and recession. If liberalism declined as a political party, its ideas lingered and mutated to include governmental responsibility to the preservation and enhancement of the conditions within which individuals flourish (Freeden, 1978; Sykes, 1997).

And in Britain, too, the advent of psychoanalysis was sometimes seen as another indication of a broad, culture-wide destabilizing trend burrowing under the fundaments of liberal society. A psychology that saw rational and measured conduct as at best a thin veneer hardly concurred with the reasonable individual actor assumed by liberalism. Charles Mercier, the Edwardian psychiatrist who combined a rationalist approach to science and a strictly juristic approach to citizenship, denounced psychoanalysis alongside spiritualism and other beliefs he saw as regressive and faddish. Psychoanalytic method, Mercier (1910) warned, blurred the lines between sanity and insanity. By delving into dreams and fantasies, psychoanalysis reduced functioning adults to incoherent delirium. By contrast, other medical professionals saw psychoanalysis as helpful for the values of personal liberty that they thought should shore up the country's democracy. Psychoanalytic theory shifted the diagnostic focus from visible conduct to the unconscious, allowing therapists to emphasize the hidden uniqueness of each person. And as psychoanalysis unearthed the bases of individual obsessions in the repression of wishes and fears, it could trace collective preoccupations such as class superiority and racism to sickness in mind and body (Hart, 1910). Freud enabled his audience to view self-reflective individuality as a dynamic trajectory that can benefit therapeutically from the external assistance of analysis. Individual agency was not a given quality. It relied on social conditions. Accordingly, medical and clinical authors who endorsed psychoanalysis tended to aggregate ideologically around advanced liberal and social-democratic positions. The psychiatrist who introduced psychoanalysis into the treatment of battled-fatigued troops during the First World War, W.H.R. Rivers, stood as a Labour candidate in the general election that followed the War. Freud's translator, James Strachey, was known to have revisionist, left-leaning sympathies (Linstrum, 2014). Wilfred Trotter (1908, 1909), an ally of Freud's primary British follower, Ernest Jones, expressed similar positions.

The pessimist and optimist accounts of liberalism's fate in the twentieth century are not necessarily incompatible. They match the same sequence of events against two different notions of what liberalism is. If liberalism simply equates with less government, then the twentieth century is characterized by its decline. But if liberalism equates with generating broader opportunities for the fulfilment of each individual and is consequently prepared to use state institutions in order to facilitate these opportunities, then the same period is one of liberal advance. Juxtaposed, the two narratives point to the substitution of a minimalist definition of political liberty by a broader and more ambitious one. Rather than facing a choice between believing a story about liberalism's decline and accepting an account of its triumph, one is looking at a chronicle of liberalism's internal transformation. If psychoanalysis features negatively in the first and affirmatively in the second, then its contents align with the broader, more interventionist idea of liberalism.

But the relationship was two-sided. To fit into a revised approach to society and the individual's place within it, psychoanalysis modified some of its own premises. As it stood, orthodox psychoanalysis was not easy to settle with a forward-looking, humanistic and interventionist social outlook. The advent of object relations theory can be understood as that modification. It proceeded primarily from analysts' clinical and professional grappling with received theory. But it was also an effort to arbitrate between Freudian theory and the revised approach to society and politics that took hold among educated professionals in Britain. In its political-theory aspect, that approach amounted to a synthesis of several liberal ideas. Read as a political theory as well, object relations thought can be understood as addressing that liberal synthesis and as dealing with the tensions and compromises among the social philosophy's constituent elements. The next section looks at the theoretical and historical makeup of the progressive, welfare-minded worldview as it crystallized in the first half of the twentieth century.

Natural Society and Individual Liberty

To transform the tenets of the veteran, age-hallowed and nationally respected liberal philosophy into a justification for the welfare state, public authors, journalists and scholars rearranged liberal theory's internal components. A crucial element of this move was a newfangled emphasis placed on an older, somewhat neglected, feature of liberal theory: the perception of individual liberty as displaying in and fulfilled through each person's ability to connect emotionally and behaviourally to others. The notion of individual sociability mediated between the various ingredients of the modified, welfare-oriented liberalism; secured liberalism against the illiberal potentialities of that combination; and allowed the resulting synthesis to be accepted as historically continuous with Britain's cherished values.

Anglophone liberalism provided two main ways for thinking about the rights people should be granted against power. The first approach was naturalist. It described rights as springing from an underlying condition that precedes all formal institutions. Naturalist liberalism is primarily associated with John Locke's seventeenth-century work. To make the case for the natural character of individual liberty, Locke had to contend with Robert Filmer's patriarchal argument, according to which humans always live in hierarchies dominated by stronger males. This is true for the family, where the father rules over women and children. It is similarly true for the state, a household-writ-large, where the king governs his subjects. Allowing a permanent entitlement to be held against the king amounts to letting children veto their parents' decisions. For Filmer, then, the very notion of embellished individual rights contradicts any social organization. To defend the constitutionalist and individualist ideology that will become liberalism, Locke (1946) answers Filmer's argument by pointing out that the household and the state differ. The first is a natural default option. The second is derivative. Reproduction, nurture and education are survival needs. As humanity would not be possible without these activities, they form the basis of universal entitlements. The social sites where they occur group into a natural society regulated by a natural law that precedes and overrides all human-made laws. Natural society may, if it so wishes, designate an enforcing agent to better guarantee that entitlements are respected, but it does not necessarily have to do so: civilizations may exist in without centralized enforcement and positive legislation. The king is merely the ruler of a political, secondary and non-natural aspect of society. He is barred from the primary, natural and free mode of shared human existence (Ryan, 2012: 460–464).

Locke, however, had to contend with another apology for absolutism, one that shared his own belief in a pre-political condition while drawing emphatically different conclusions from it. Associated mainly with Thomas Hobbes, this second absolutist perspective saw the natural condition as violent. In the absence of a central authority, each person caters for themselves, managing threats from others by killing or fleeing. The state of nature leaves no room for anything but the struggle for survival. Neither knowledge nor culture is possible. To avoid such a miserable existence, Hobbes suggests, individuals transfer their capacity of self-defence to a sovereign who controls all means of coercion. Being all-powerful, the sovereign neutralizes the mutual fear that permeated individuals' lives prior to the establishment of sovereignty. One's neighbour is as powerless as oneself. The struggle ceases. Production, trade, arts and crafts commence. Society originates in political power. There can be no argument from a natural society against the absolute ruler (Manent, 1995: 20–38; Ryan, 2012: 411–452).

To counter Hobbes, Locke appeals to what he sees as humans' constitutive, divinely ordained need to associate with each other. The formation of the family and the village is powered by the drive to interact with others that, Locke (1946) thinks, underlies sexuality, parenting and commerce alike. Desire for pleasure and gain are that drive's aids and expressions rather than its causes. The basic human units are essentially peaceful, as they are self-regulated by their participants' interest in preserving the occasion for sociability to unfold. As sociability instils a wish in each person to be validated by another person, natural society is fundamentally, if never practically, egalitarian. While they are hierarchic and given to differences of interest, its units are not made to gratify one participant at the expenses of the other. Despite this peaceful character, however, different households or villages might have existentially contradicting interests that cannot be mitigated by the quest for company. To avoid violence, the occupants of natural society may contract into a political society and generate the organs of state. By signing into the social contract, participants establish an additional, political sphere, where the natural functions of parents, offspring, employers and workers are suspended, while individuals all assume the equal and identical persona of the citizen. Locke's monarchist opponents, patriarchal and contractual alike, saw the social world as unified: the state held authority over the entirety of its citizens' lives. By contrast, Locke's liberal world divides into two realms: helpless children are raised in homes where parents instruct them, while responsible adults inhabit the world of civic deliberation and law as well as that of privacy, friendship and primary ties. The father is not king as he has no lethal power over his children. The king is not father as his authority depends on the consent of adult citizens. This split landscape is entailed by the English Bill of Rights as it is by the American Constitution. It resided at the core of liberalism until the end of the nineteenth century (Manent, 1995: 39–52).

But it was not left unchallenged. Alternative forms of liberalism emerged in the centuries that succeeded Locke's intervention. Utilitarianism was one of them. Late eighteenth-century utilitarians thought that all institutions rely on balances of pain and pleasure rather than on the consent of naturally free individuals. Appeals to nature for justifying any particular institution serve the vested interests of whoever benefits from these institutions. Hence, utilitarianism rejects Locke's account of natural liberty. Reworking utilitarianism at the middle of the nineteenth century, John Stuart Mill retained the notion of utility as the measure of all institutions, alongside the older utilitarian dislike of invoking nature for legitimizing these institutions. However, unlike earlier utilitarians, Mill argued that utility is not a calculable, objective quality. An unbearable agony for one person may be an experience worthy of one's time for another. Utility should be instead based on every separate person's chosen life-ends. The polity should organize to allow each person to go their own way in pursuit of these ends, as long as their actions do not infringe on others. Like Locke, then, Mill founds a liberal settlement organized around entitlements that protect individual autonomy. But for the natural rights derived from the functions of home and village, Mill substitutes a right to follow one's personal project, conditioned on avoiding harm to others. Subsequently, the boundaries of privacy and politics move away from where Locke had drawn them. As life-projects differ, the means for pursuing them differ too: some people fulfil themselves in family and trade, others by adventure, sports or scholarship. As liberty resides in each individual's own choices rather than in performing specific actions within set sites, then that liberty can be impinged upon by other individuals within these sites, as well as by government.

The family household made by the Bill of Rights immune to governmental power might crush its weaker members and compromise their liberty. Protection from such impingement can only be provided by government, establishing the state's legitimate intervention within the region Locke had deemed private. Children, for example, should be shielded by the state from parental decisions that compromised their futures (Ryan, 2012: 695–728).

Realist critics of liberal philosophy equated its historical variants with a rationalist belief in progress that allows reason to dissolve all tensions, thus ending by denying any space for contingency, risk, and decision, or, in other words, for politics itself (Morgenthau, 1946). The allegation has some merit because liberals like Locke and Mill were interested in maximizing individual liberty and therefore sought to confine and constrain government while relying on rationalist arguments. They may hereby create the impression that they wish to place an interlocking, benevolent ideal of reason in the space where conflict and decision-making were. However, both Locke and Mill draw a line beyond which the interactions, rights and dynamics of individuality cease, and a realm of shared public action begins. They draw it in different places but retain the essential separation of civic politics from private life. Historical liberalism, therefore, can be optimistic about the ability of reason to limit danger and violence, but this optimism is guarded and reserved. As differing from the pastoralist visions of patriarchal communitarians or radical socialists, liberalism involves conceding that our existence includes irreducible breaks and divisions: without such a possibility, the notion of personal freedom itself would not make sense as all people would be expected to conduct themselves in accordance with universal precepts.

However, as if to vindicate the realist, the early twentieth century effort to combine several liberal philosophies so as to allow liberalism to expand did involve the consequence of challenging the autonomy of politics and its distinction from privacy. Liberalism's turn towards welfare in the early twentieth century involved combining Locke and Mill and aligning both with the period's scientific concepts. Early twentieth-century authors like L.T. Hobhouse (1904: 134–135) argued that individual differentiation is grounded in an evolutionary biology that hands the edge over to species in which each individual is distinct from, while being capable of being intensely close to, and peacefully engaging with, the next one:

> The evolution which has created man, which has engendered human society and developed civilisation out of barbarism, is…not based upon the struggle for existence, but upon an opposed principle by which the struggle for existence is gradually subdued, a principle of peace rather than war, of co-operation rather than competition, of love rather than hate.

Hence, rights for a private space with both individual differentiation and the capacity to associate with others are mandated by nature. That space includes the family and the household, which should be left independent from institutions and politics. However, as the nature to which rights are anchored is evolutionary rather than static, individual liberty should also be seen as involving creativity. Utilized differently by each person, freedom generates a greater pool of ideas. A free society, then, should protect its members not just by immunizing specific sites such as the family, but also by assuring the discretion of each individual within those sites. The Millian, utilitarian right to do whatever does not harm others merges with the Lockean right to perform specific actions within a stable private sphere. This combination allowed twentieth-century liberals to demand the expansion of rights from life, liberty and property, over to education, medical care, accommodation and employment. Rendered categorical by their basis in nature, such rights justified governmental intervention in arenas like the workplace and the market in order to enhance individual autonomy within them. The expansion of government's role from a minimalist foreman to proactive guarantor and provider became possible from liberal grounds (Clarke, 1978; Freeden, 1978).

However, this compound of liberal strands was conceptually vulnerable. Its philosophical constituents largely retained the sphere division. But when these constituents were combined, the sphere division weakened. Locke distinguished politics from privacy in order to refute the undifferentiated worlds of Filmer and Hobbes, where governmental power stopped nowhere. Mill kept the divide by separating acts that impact the actor alone and thus fall within the realm of privacy, from those that impact others and are thus made accessible to public power. The sphere boundary is retained by both authors, if in different locations. But when Mill is fused with Locke, that boundary blurs. Because of Mill, the utilitarian component of the synthesis emphasizes that harm to their separate members' liberty can be wrought within all social sites. Because of Locke, the naturalist component arms the need to protect liberty by intervening in social sites with an imperative quality: not enforcing rights to education or working hours infringes on a universal, naturally given morality that precedes human legislation. As a result of the fusion between the naturalist and utilitarian elements, the political invasion of privacy might turn mandatory and boundless. As government is the instrument of natural liberty, there can be no appeal against it to that liberty.

As Hobhouse's reference to love as the organizing social principle illustrates, the advanced liberals of the early twentieth century replied to this potential danger by emphasizing anew, and drawing additional conclusions from, Locke's notion of innate sociability. For Locke, sociability establishes and defines natural society. The desire for company generates the various family, village and commerce-oriented units that inhabit the private realm. But sociability has limits: beyond family and village, one is bound at some point to encounter strangers to whom one is not committed by friendship and its more distant inflections in collegiate relationships and partnership. The encounter might turn violent. A society of strangers may choose to contract into political society and interpose an impersonal authority between its members. While overall accepting this account, early twentieth-century reforming liberals suggested that the setting had changed from the early-modern one. Locke thought that sociability always encounters limits that encourage the formation of political society because the communication channels he envisaged were still underdeveloped. Early-moderns could form a sociable, essentially peaceful bond with a limited number of others. By contrast, in the complex industrial civilization of late modernity, interpersonal communication does not necessarily meet any final frontier. The sociable motivation can be expressed through venues that develop all the time. The benevolence of natural society may therefore expand into further arenas, including those that had earlier been strictly impersonal. Political and civic activity may be permeated by the fundamental sociability of the private sphere. Instead of being a merely coercive organ keeping watch over the otherwise self-regulating natural society, government may become another site where people communicate and cooperate (Hobhouse, 1994: 35–36). Under such changed conditions, governmental concern with the home, as in providing for the education and even the feeding of young school children, was not necessarily an invasion of the intimate sphere by a rationale foreign to it. It was instead the institutional expression of natural society's increasing hold over public affairs.

Sociability's fundamental role and its potentially expansive reach were thus functional for allaying the fears that the fusion of Locke and Mill might unleash an alienated bureaucracy on society. Reforming liberals repeatedly emphasized the ubiquity of company-seeking behaviour. For Hobhouse (1924: 151), human conduct is shaped by the quest for validation. The individual mind, he writes, 'is inherently a centre of relationships to others, and craves these relationships if it does not find them'. Aggression and domination illustrate the inescapability of this drive rather than negate it because they show the dependence of the aggressor on the responses of the victim. At society's irreducible core, the search for meaningful validation structures the family. The burden of childcare is made desirable and endurable by the joy parents experience (Hobhouse, 1921: 34–35). That joy derives from the fulfilment of the parents' sociable drive, which is installed by evolution for that very purpose. As the home is based on the need for company, the role of physical sexuality is relatively demoted. As in Locke, desire becomes a channel for the underlying sociability. The 'sex impulse', Hobhouse (1924: 158) writes, 'is no more than a bodily need or appetite' that borrows its significance from its collaboration with the 'impulse to give and seek response'. Sociability has in principle no ultimate, fixed boundary. Unlike sex, the motivations of friendship and concern for others can find outlets beyond the household without endangering the household itself. Activities based on these needs may reach out to encompass the entire society, while retaining the home as their essential hub. Parental and filial emotions, Hobhouse (1924: 151) writes, are the 'the prime examples of an impulse inherent in mind, and potentially as wide as the range of life'.

A commonwealth conditioned by the emotions arising from the experiences of family and friendship builds institutions that provide for the private realm where these experiences occur rather than intrude on it. This perception underlies the comprehensive welfare-state programme formulated from liberal premises during the Second World War. William Beveridge, who is largely identified with that plan, asserted that guaranteeing the home's stability is legitimately a state concern, because the care of spouses and parents is a fundamental human need and therefore forms the bedrock of a universal entitlement (Beveridge, 1942: 139–140; 1948: 238–243). 'Family life', Beveridge (1942: 43–44) writes, 'its responsibilities and its cares, are the material of which most of human happiness...is made'. Providing environmental guarantees for the home's viability and for parental functioning, securing ample food and clothing, and allowing a minimum of job security are all means for attaining these ends. As the quest for relating and for company expands to shape further contacts and associations, respecting it as a natural trait through which people fulfil themselves entails recognizing, encouraging and enabling the multiple sites where it can unfold. Individuality expresses itself through engagement in voluntary groups, trade partnerships, shared artistic ventures and scholarly debate. Personal freedom registers as engaging in activities with new associates and additional types of relationships, generating a plural society made of overlapping voluntary associations (Beveridge, 1948: 319–320). Government is an aid to this expanding sphere of human bonds which is ultimately as broad as humanity itself (Hobhouse, 1922: 235).

The protected private realm thus exceeds the home and any other static location: all social arenas can be occasions for individuality to display itself by communicating with others. While expressing the characters of Locke's natural society, such a perception is also compatible with Mill's notion of liberty as space for pursuing subjectively defined ends. The profit motive retains its legitimacy as a vehicle for the expression of individual wishes. It is however placed in a derivative, inferior position relative to the sociable impulse. While allowed to stand, the market should be curbed when it harms people's ability to have a fulfilling home life or develop interests outside the home. This might happen when long working hours leave no leisure for family members to interact beyond the necessities of food and reproduction. It might similarly occur when dependence on the caprice of employers and landlords tars all encounters with anxiety. With this outlook at his background, the progressive educator and social scientist, Graham Wallas (1914: 373) could suggest gearing the social-policy apparatus towards rescuing social isolates by granting them leisure and public spaces for meeting others. The combined perception of liberty expects government to counteract economic forces. It similarly tasks the state with creating opportunities for all to engage with others (Goodin, 1988: 70–71).

Ethics and National Identity

Beyond mediating the internal tension in advanced liberalism's political theory, the centrality accorded by early twentieth-century British reformers to sociability served other intellectual and cultural ends. Throughout the nineteenth century, British thinkers grappled with the necessity of adhering to the secular and individualist tone of enlightenment while escaping its mechanical and alienated implications. Such alienation could take the form of a harsh capitalism in which only measurable productivity mattered. To avoid such results, many Victorian and Edwardian thinkers attempted to create a secular ethics that would be grounded in social practices instead of appealing to a declining religion. T.H. Green taught that the friendly encounter with and commitment to the other was the chief educative experience. Within this mode of thought, individuals are never complete or satisfied on their own: they unceasingly cluster together to be morally, intellectually and emotionally enriched through interaction with their fellows. Acting with and for others is normatively higher and ultimately more satisfying than acting solely for oneself (Collini, 1991; den Otter, 1996; Nicholson, 1990).

However, for the source of their perceptions, Green and likeminded thinkers relied to differing degrees on Hegel, for whom the need for recognition drives a tense dialectic of hostility and commitment that creates ever larger social units. Hegel cast the simplest and most common human bonds, those of sexual and romantic partners and those of parents and children, as necessary for the construction of a broader order that ties together emotion and obligation. Emotion and desire were the educative tools that concretized one's dependence on and indebtedness to others. The indebtedness grew with the scope of social bonds. Conjugal partners exchange gifts, thereby symbolizing their readiness to sacrifice for each other. The last, ultimate bond was that of citizen and state. Here, individuals were called upon for giving the ultimate gift, that of life, as a measure of their realizing their sociable, recognition-seeking nature. Hegel, accordingly, places the state beyond any censure or law outside itself. The state was an ultimate, if never final, embodiment of humans' social character (Brooks, 2007). Unsurprisingly, this conclusion fed into the political hostility that British public opinion, including many of its intellectuals, felt towards Germany in the twentieth century's first decades. Hegel's advocacy of the state's unquestioned authority seemed to be the source of the militarism and aggression displayed by Prussia and its successors (Bradley, 1979). If Hegel's observation about the role of recognition was valuable, it attached to a dialectical, essentially violent view of history that British reformers could not endorse without modification.

The search for a principle of social cohesion that did not impinge on liberty and individuality and avoided establishing an unaccountable collective organ took many forms. There were those who looked back to the Greek spirit of civil friendship; and there were those who longed for the intimate medieval hearth (Burns, 1919; Nicklin, 1898). The progressive liberals' device of relying on evolution to connect Locke and Mill was another such attempt. It held the advantage over similar projects by having behind it the pedigree of British liberalism itself, in the form of its eminent historical thinkers, alongside a scientific discipline then at the height of its prestige. As opposed to Hegelian dialectic, the sociable drive fulfilled by marriage and childcare harboured no residual tension and demanded no ultimate sacrifice. The political settlement it fitted into was liberal and democratic rather than statist and absolutist.

The appeal to sociability also created a commonality between advanced liberals and the wider public, a commonality sometimes missing from high-minded social reform movements. The simple pleasures of family life and childcare were a consensual symbol for the British public of the early twentieth century, when various commentators of differing political hues compared the English household favourably with what they saw as its more disciplinarian and formalist Continental counterparts (Harris, 1993: 79–84, 93–94). Converting this widespread belief in the superiority of the supportive, caring and tolerant home to its harsher counterpart into a generalizing statement on its evolutionary worth, Hobhouse (1911: 25) writes that 'the family in which parental love is strongest will have an advantage in competition with other families'. This perception of the home as a favoured site for personal expression and fulfilment and at the same time a source of collective pride and strength could easily be synthesized with the new emphasis on a sociability as compatible with individual worth. The compound outlook respected both the locally cherished ideal of the loving family and the idea of individual liberty, an equally important source of national distinction. The outcome was a view of human attachment as both functional for survival needs and respecting personal freedom while also having the most familiar, everyday sites of home, family and conjugal ties as its main locus.

By highlighting sociability as the core human trait at the basis of individual entitlements, advanced liberalism pre-empted the risks harboured by the synthesis of Locke and Mill. Pervaded by the genuine interest in retaining meaningful communication with others, the private sphere which is the locus of liberty becomes peaceful and benevolent. As the sociable motivation is expansive and creative, it crosses the boundary of the home and the village outwards in order to inform all other relationships, including those that connect citizens. Government is encumbered with preserving and enabling this process and is, in turn, shaped by it. The policy product of this perception is a welfare regime that provides for a society made of free, creative and mutually interacting individuals, rather than acting as a sovereign ruler split away from natural society and arbitrarily governing it.

Liberal Psychoanalysis

The revised liberal perspective shared some features with classical psychoanalysis. While not always relying explicitly on Freud, reforming authors were on the look for an innovative, humanistic and developmental account of the mind (Tolman, 1987). A psychology that takes into account the idiosyncratic experiences, memories and sensibilities of each individual person appealed to advanced liberals. Such a psychology could define humans as exceeding the determination of blind biological or economic forces. At the same time, the accessibility of each person to a method of psychological enquiry also meant that humans were not inherently chaotic or irrational. For Freud, the rational adulthood of work, legal accountability and civic obligation was shaped by the baggage carried over from the early-family setting. For progressive liberals, responsible individual agency was an environmental product and was rooted in one's upbringing and access to an equitable choice of opportunities. Moreover, as the Edwardian and interwar author John Hobson noted, Freud's theory showed that human behaviour was not reducible to instrumental rationality. The mind included components of spontaneity and creativity that exceeded, and sometimes challenged, the social order: a democracy seeking to respect its citizens was obliged to tolerate, and even encourage, the wide array of these citizens' perceptions and behaviour, tolerating even rebellious conduct as one of its legitimate constituents (Gerson, 2004: 87–88).

However, the interface between orthodox psychoanalysis and revised liberalism presented its own problems. For Freud, the private, interior existence that percolates into the world of work and public affairs is not unambiguously benign. Freud describes a child who is primarily narcissistic and a psyche that is constantly disrupted by the effects of competition for inherently scarce resources. Reasonable functioning entails repressing aggression and desire, like a foreign garrison controlling a hostile populace. One's innermost wishes contradict each other and are essentially incompatible with the social order. If the oedipal situation is society's bedrock, nothing in that society can avoid envy and aggression. Freud's dislike of social perfectionism grew more intense with the introduction of the death drive into his theory in the interwar period. As human ties involve frustration, they elicit aggression. Social units temporarily resolve the problem by directing the aggression outwards, against other units. The bigger and more internally organized the unit, the more voluminous the frustration and incipient violence stored within it. When reaching the organizational level of entire states, violence becomes lethal, with destructive wars fought to maintain internal cohesion. Such violence employs the death drive as its tool, but as that drive is independent, it cannot be wholly regulated by institutions. War erupts because of the scarcity of gratification, but would still occur if all needs were met. Any programme that upholds an essentially better future as a realistic option is harmful: it merely postpones, and by doing so ultimately amplifies, the tensions it desires to reduce. Consequently, Freud aligns with Hobbes rather than with Locke or Mill. Freud's reduction of justice and law to power relations undermines any idea of objective justice and inalienable human rights, and engenders, in his turn, more elaborations of Hobbesian political theory (Brunner, 2000; Schuett, 2007).

The dangers to any project of liberal and democratic reform involved in accepting Freud's theory were openly noted by British liberals. While commending Freud for offering a broader, more dynamic and potentially developmental perception of the mind, Hobson (1921: 44–45) was also aware that Freud recognized no rational organizing principle in society and could accordingly undermine any sustained, principle attempt at improvement:

> The Freudian psycho-analysis, spreading like wildfire among continental intellectuals, had already begun to reach this country and to complete the demolition of the claim of man to be a reasoning animal. Science and reason were to be put in their proper place as tools for the creative soul of man, whose pulsing instincts, emotions, intuitions and desires were the real determinants of human conduct (including the discovery and systematization of knowledge) and were inciting us to mould the physical and spiritual universe according to our hearts desire.

The reforming, social-minded liberalism of which Hobson was one of the main advocates was, as earlier noted, synchronized with many of its environment's sensibilities. The search of an educated, socially conscientious elite for a secular ethics based on real-world engagement combined with a broader perception of British society as pervaded by a warm and tolerant, if usually implicit, view of the family household. Expressly political authors were therefore voicing concerns that were shared by many others. If they were taxed for accommodating a malleable and dynamic individual personality with an overall peaceful and lawful perception of society, so were these others. These included the doctors and psychiatrists who coalesced into the object relations school. Their psychoanalytical theory modifies Freud in accordance with these concerns.

Object relations theorists were not primarily political authors and had little to do with the conceptual struggles of liberalism. However, several factors make their worldview align with reforming liberal thought. Object relations theory's premises render it more interested than other analytic variants in the concrete, living practices of society. By abandoning the seduction hypothesis, Freud was left with mainly intra-psychic factors to account for the oedipal situation and its consequences. Departing from Freud by investigating an earlier stage of development, Klein retained Freud's focus on perceptions and fantasies. The child's innate aggression and the child's concepts of persecuting objects stood at the centre of her model. If the mother performed as an anchor for the child's conflicting instincts by being a real and whole object, that anchor was needed in order to stabilize the internal world that still constituted the theory's focus. In the form of the always-present paranoid position, that internal world continues to effect adult life. By contrast to both Freud and Klein, object relations authors pay more attention to observable childhood: to how the mother holds the child, to the games child and parent play, and to the tangible setting of the home. Bowlby and Winnicott, in particular, note the tangible interactions of children and parents. The British school is consequently more interested than orthodox or Kleinian analyses were in the external world.

Additionally, object relations theory includes an inherent ideological factor. Psychoanalysis shares with most liberal philosophies a methodological and normative concern with individuality. This contributes to Freud's earlier-mentioned criticism of utopian thought: health and functioning differ for each person and can only be achieved by conversing with their internal worlds. They cannot be imposed from without by a collectivity. The British analysts retain this position. Like Freud, they repeatedly disapprove of ideological purism. Ian Suttie (1933) perceives the doctrinaire forms of capitalism and socialism alike as pathologies that arise from emotional deficits. Fairbairn echoes by describing totalitarianism as an ultimately futile attempt to recapture the symbiotic, reassuring intimacy of the first bond. Dictatorships that cast their leaders as fathers of their nations and brothers of their citizens infantilize their subjects and hamper their healthy, gradual distancing from the family setting. Fairbairn (1952: 79–83) views democracy as representing an adult ability to hold one's need for company alongside the inevitability of separation. Regardless of object relations theory's upbeat notion of the first relationship, these reservations about the pretensions of comprehensive ideology echo Freud's suspicions. Individuals minds differ. Their aspirations and the conditions within which they can sense fulfilment cannot be reduced to a social scheme or conform to a preset pattern. There can be no unmitigated and perpetual bliss.

Combining the focus on individuals and the dismissal of utopian ideology while still wishing to transcend Freud's gloom, object relations theory arrives at a worldview that is compatible with welfare-oriented liberalism. The affiliation is systemic, exceeding the obvious convergence of both analysts and political philosophers on the need for holding and social provision. One measure of that affiliation is that object relations theory offers something akin to Locke's notion of a natural society held together by an inborn sociable drive, which contrasts with the views offered by Hobbes – and Freud – of a society based on essentially self-regarding, primarily narcissistic individuals. The perception elaborated by object relations theorists renders personal relationships empowering and peaceful and allows them to infiltrate the public world, but it also entails that this benevolence cannot be accurately reproduced by political institutions.

The suggestion of a default-option healthy society is already apparent in Ian Suttie's contributions. Written in the 1920s and early 1930s, Ian Suttie's works are prevalently regarded as an early variant of object relations theory. Along with his wife and occasional co-author, Jane Suttie, Ian Suttie explicitly aimed to offer a comprehensive alternative to Freud's deadlocked and forlorn worldview. Freud, Ian Suttie thinks, generalizes from illness, presenting an abnormality as an unavoidable normality, and demanding that we accept the brunt of a sick civilization while abjectly thanking the tyranny that oppresses us for holding chaos at bay. As an alternative, Ian Suttie offers a psychology geared to make environmental betterment possible. To do this, Ian Suttie revises Freud's perception of the first, formative experiences, and consequently generates an account of the natural condition. Playing Locke to Freud's Hobbes, Ian Suttie (1999) suggests that caring relationships precede competition for sensuous, material satisfaction. In infancy, which is humans' earliest environment, libidinal gratification has as yet little survival value. Company, however, does have that value, as without an attending adult infants do not live to reproductive adulthood (19). Ian Suttie and Jane Suttie (1932a: 104–105) argue that while food, warmth and shelter may be furnished by a parent, that parent's presence has first to be secured. As the first imperative, the wish to retain the mother's proximity conditions individuals throughout their lives to seek and maintain human contact. Its forms change through childhood. From keeping the mother concerned solely with the child, the child advances to learn how to gain her attention for shared pursuits and objects, such as songs and pictures. When this is achieved, the child is able to draw others, besides the mother, into common interests. Peers are engaged with through games, music and shared meals. Art, sports, science – and civilization itself – are all variant consequences of this core drive to seek company (Suttie, 1999: 16). '[T]he whole of life', Suttie (1933: 162) writes, 'comes to fill the void the mother once filled'. Society is held together by the mutually interested and therefore peaceful, sociable drive of its members. It exists prior to any organ of coercion or political institution.

The predominance of the sociable impetus entails that other motivations occupy a relatively secondary role, leading to a different hierarchy of motives than the one described by Freud. Suttie and Suttie (1932b: 204–210) accordingly play down libido and aggression. On its own, sexual desire is no more significant than other functions that relieve the body of surplus inputs or contents. What grants sexuality its emotional charge is its capacity to use the body as a transmission device aimed at relating to others. Aggression, for its part, is not an essential human feature at all. It is instead an aberration that stems from flaws in maternal attention, a deficit that the individual experiences as resentment. To compensate for this, and to regain the ability to relate, the child devises strategies that include attempts to control or destroy the mother. These patterns of relating are later projected onto society at large and cause social malaise (Suttie, 1999: 52–53).

Ian Suttie's early death cut his project short in the mid-1930s. His expressly ideological criticism of Freud was rarely repeated with the same pitch within the British school. But the notion of sociability as humanity's essential, natural feature, was further elaborated by the school's later authors. The implications of sociability's primacy for psychoanalytic theory were explored in the 1930s by Fairbairn. Clinical, rather than ideological concerns compelled Fairbairn (1952: 84–85) to seek explanations for the failures of therapeutic interventions based on classical psychoanalysis. Some patients could not be reached by Freudian methodology or accounted for by Freudian theory. Attempting to resolve the riddle, Fairbairn suggested that orthodox analysis's blind spot was early infancy, a time dominated by a different order of priorities than the one that structures the already verbal oedipal stage. At the top of that order stands the relationship with the primary caretaker rather than a competition with a third agent who intrudes on that relationship. Perceived or real disruptions to the relationship with the mother register as fissures in the personality. Fairbairn superimposed a map of these splits over Freud's taxonomy of id, ego and superego.

Unavoidable failures of maternal attention elicit resentment, while the mother's presence excites and arouses. To manage this complexity, the infant splits the representation of the mother into three objects. The rejecting object stands for the resentment caused by perceived or real maternal neglect. Relationship with this object is characterized by doses of aggression and abject docility, and is taken up by a split-off rejecting ego. The exciting aspect of the mother is similarly broken off and met by a libidinal part-ego. A central, non-aggressive and desexualized part object remains, with which a central part-ego engages in an idealizing relationship (Fairbairn, 1952: 82–136). The rejecting ego which attacks the self parallels Freud's idea of a ferocious superego. The libidinal ego that tantalizes with desire corresponds to Freud's notion of the id. The central approving ego matches Freud's idea of the ego. The discomfort that produces the splits is not caused by scarcity but by the relationship with the object, which appears to repudiate and attract the infant at the same time (119–125, 135–136). The entire personality, then, is organized to meet the primary imperative of relating to the mother. The psyche's internal parts are condensed images of maternal aspects and the child's position relative to them.

Fairbairn (1952) uses this insight to reinterpret another classical map, that of erotogenic stages. Material motivations that are experienced by the individual's body alone are deemphasized in his scheme, while the formative significance of relationship is played up. Body sensations carry messages, but do not provide these messages' contents. Communication is channelled through the body's surface, the sensitivity of which intensifies with the child's age. This transformation begins with the oral phase, in which communication is localized, relatively simple and consists in taking what the environment has to offer. Gradually, the child advances into the more complex genital phase, in which the emphasis is on exchange and response. At all stages, corporeal sensation is a means rather than an end of communication. At the oral phase, for example, the thumb stands for the mother rather than functioning as a mass of flesh that happens to be available for the stimulation of the mouth (34–35). The individual is interested not so much in balancing a closed economy of bodily sensations as in interacting with a significant other. Freud's and Karl Abraham's cartography of stimuli, Fairbairn writes, 'is based upon a failure to recognize that the function of libidinal pleasure is essentially to provide a sign-post to the object' (33). Communication precedes and conditions the organization of the body into a distinct whole that has particular desires (Hughes, 2000: 251–254). Ian Suttie and Fairbairn differ on the level of disruption that can be normally expected within the first relationship, with Suttie being more optimistic, but they converge in perceiving that relationship as a template and a springboard for later life: all social sites are permeated by the templates acquired within an early, supportive and caring environment. A natural, underlying mode of interaction exists prior to all institutions and laws.

Other analysts delved further into this naturalist streak, echoing Ian Suttie's reliance on evolutionary biology. Based initially on his observations of child-rearing during the havoc of the Second World War, John Bowlby came to see maternal presence and the stability of the home as critical for health. To this, Bowlby added a comparative methodology and a biologically informed perspective. Like Suttie, Bowlby (1973: 29) suggests importing a Darwinian perspective into psychology as a corrective to the metaphysical character of Freud's approach. Complex animals can only survive their first years with the help of others. Surveying researches from various disciplines, Bowlby suggests that such species employ a thermostat-like control system that sends off warning signals when proximity to others falls below a certain level. This system conditions the young animal's behaviour, shapes the adult specimen and moulds the conduct of the species as a whole. Like these species, humans are also impacted by the role of attachment as the first concern and the first urge. The various shapes that satisfying it takes constitute civilization: nature, understood literally as biology, places humans in a position where their basic requirement is company. They cope by configuring their environments to yield it (Bowlby, 1997: 37–57).

The perception of sociability as the basis of all other psychic and social dynamics is repeated by Donald Winnicott. Initially close to Klein, Winnicott was not particularly enthusiastic about importing biological vocabularies into psychoanalysis and may therefore not seem to be an obvious candidate for supporting a naturalist take. Nonetheless, Winnicott (1984) joins Suttie, Fairbairn and Bowlby in asserting that at the original point from which all humans start, a society and its interpersonal relationships already exist. In that setting, Winnicott insists, there is no such thing as an isolated specimen: '[I]f you show me a baby you certainly show me also someone caring for the baby, or at least a pram with someone's eyes and ears glued to it. One sees a "nursing couple"' (99). The lack of individual separateness in the initial stages of life goes beyond the fact of physical dependence. It involves the absence of inner cohesion. The neonate is an aggregate of sensations and body parts without an organizing principle. 'At this very early stage', Winnicott (1988: 131) writes, 'it is not logical to think in terms of an individual...because there is not yet an individual self there'. The internal organization of the child has to be enabled and supported by the attention of the parent who is holding the child physically, and whose presence functions as an external perimeter that contains the various stimuli and orders them into a meaningful whole. Relationship, again, precedes individuality and enables it (Winnicott, 1965b: 88, 1989: 568). A structured group with roles and functions such as those of child and parent is already present where humans start. The other concepts we deploy – the continuities of time and space, the cohesion of our own selves as distinct from our environment – are derivative. In its natural condition, humanity is already grouped into units and its driving motivations governed by the need to relate.

This perception of naturally evolved and universal sociability as founding a society regulated by the complementarity of roles places object relations theory close to Locke. It hints that we do not owe our lives to commands and positive laws but to a universal, shared drive to associate. Unlike the tortured individuals of Freud's outlook, we are not necessarily designed to endlessly repress ourselves and fight others. The home, the care of children it provides and the sociable attitude it upholds are primary, making them normatively superior to, and potentially carriers of rights to be held against, formal institutions. An autonomous private sphere is established, lending object relations theory a closeness to the early-modern foundation of British constitutional liberalism.

Creative Privacy

There is, however, a significant difference between the natural society assumed by Locke and the one implied by the analysts. In Locke, natural society never changes. Its stability contrasts with a civic, political sphere where decisions on new situations and emergencies call for deliberation and innovative solutions. Nature dictates the roles of father and mother, parent and child. Born powerless, humans gradually acquire the ability to shoulder the demands of work and parenting. They similarly acquire the mental powers of rational thinking that qualify them for membership in the social contract. These powers are akin to teeth: invisible at birth, they are always there and would invariably assume their final shape within a known period. Nurture, accordingly, involves little conscious agency, and has a definite termination point. Politics and the civic realm, by contrast, are inhabited by rational adults who have agency and use that agency to induce change. But as we have natural rights, politics is barred from the private, natural, realm, where the family lives. We can argue about war and peace, but not about parents' responsibility and authority over their children.

In relations-based psychoanalysis, by contrast, the early-infancy setting that occupies the same place as the state of nature does in Locke's scheme exhibits more dynamic characters. Attachment itself is universal, as it is essential for survival. Its pattern, however, is mutable, moulding each individual into a unique personality. Different parents react differently to children's needs, generating varying attachment styles that become the bases of different individual and cultural forms. Suttie and Suttie (1932b) write that the mother's constant presence provides the child with a stable anchor among inchoate sensations. At the same time, this presence teaches the child about the existence of a distinct and separate other, as the child is shown that the mother is another person who is independent from the child. Parental responses can generate varying levels of separateness and individuality. When mothers see motherhood as their one asset, they become subtly dependent on their children, and transmit this sense of dependence to these children. The ensuing adult personality would be less confident about its own agency, and would seek to control others while being more prone to domination by others. How the family behaves produces different outcomes: it is not uniformly determined by biological functions.

Bowlby (1997: 265–330) goes further into the mechanism through which attachment generates variations in individual and culture. While the infant is born with an impersonal drive to socialize that is indistinguishable from the behavioural apparatus of any other neonate, the child develops a particular identity by attaching to a particular other. Governed by the evolutionary imperative to seek company, the infant in its first weeks of life responds to any human face. With time, the empty template of sociability is filled with a specific attachment figure, normally the biological mother. The particular mode of maintaining proximity to her is determined by her response and by environmental factors. The pattern of attachment contains within it a range of possibilities, of which the emergence of the healthy and confident adult personality is one. That possibility is realized when the mother's presence lends the child a secure basis from which to explore. Maternal care creates the temporal continuity that allows the child to conceptualize a future over which the child may have some leverage: thought is causally related to action, action to consequence (Bowlby, 1951: 55). The more securely attached, the further the child would venture beyond the range limited by immediate contact with the mother, having internalized the security her attention provides. Through early nurture, Bowlby (52) writes, 'we become less and less at the mercy of our immediate environment and of its impact upon us, and more and more able to pursue our own goals...and to select and create our own environment'. Care builds up different levels of confidence, while attention produces individually varying ability to do without attention (Holmes, 1993: 70–71). The rational subject is enabled by a specific configuration of the home and the community of which the home is a part. It is not predictably given.

The control exerted over the range of adult behaviours by differing parental responses is also central to Winnicott's thought. The achievement of the capacity for distinct autonomy involves realizing one's irretrievable separation from, and limited power over, others. What is lost with separation is referred to by Winnicott (1988: 106–107) as the illusion of omnipotence – an illusion that is nonetheless essential for the very process of overcoming it. Personal development begins with immediate and constant parental attention. The parent responds to the child's wishes for comfort, food and warmth. From the infant's point of view there is no gap between desire and fulfilment, as the wish is immediately granted. The world is continuous with the child's own wishes. Delay and frustration, which are necessary if personal differentiation is to take place, are experienced as disillusionment about the parent's unconditional availability. To withstand separation, the child has to believe in the mother's eventual return. The mother should be perceived as a separate entity, of which the child has a clear internal representation steadfastly kept even in her absence (Winnicott, 1984: 221–228). At this point the child can create what Winnicott calls the transitional object. The reassuring internal representation of the mother is projected onto a tangible item, such as a blanket or a soft toy, to which the child ascribes special meaning and identity. The transitional object helps the child bridge parental unavailability (229–234). That object is simultaneously internal and external: it carries subjective meaning, but, being tangible, it is also objectively perceived. In later life, the soft toy or blanket is substituted by games, artistic creativity and intellectual discussion. Such activities provide individuals with spaces where they can externalize their psychic contents and make them available for conversation and play. These activities and the associations based on them vary as the modes of interaction differ from every family setting to the next (Winnicott, 1991: 95–103).

Conjointly, then, Ian Suttie, Jane Suttie, Bowlby and Winnicott describe the nurturing activity that meets the child's needs as universally natural and as allowing the formation of the confident and explorative adult personality. A natural and naturally benign society is available, and is made of distinct individuals. However, child-rearing is vulnerable, which necessitates psychology's own function. If their trust in the benevolent operation of the home places object relations thinkers close to Locke, their professional perception of the family as requiring counsel nudges them closer to Mill. The mature individual persona does not hatch in a universally identical form from the parental chrysalis, as Locke had imagined. To be capable of autonomy, to enjoy liberty, the human individual requires, and merits, environmental provision (Nussbaum, 2006: 391–392). The maturation process does not unfold predictably and uniformly. Rational individuality ceases to be a given feature. It becomes an ideal, a measure of the home's ability to assure the conditions where the sense of chronological continuity and spatial contiguity can form. As individuality is malleable and vulnerable, it requires protection. Such protection includes fostering the conditions under which individuality can be nurtured. As a stable household is beneficial for the nurture patterns that establish individual autonomy and agency, that household merits not only the respite from the public's discretion as embodied in the rights to a sheltered privacy, but also help and counsel that may be provided by that public. While guaranteed against arbitrary intervention, the household can legitimately become an object of societal concern and exert a legitimate claim to services and assistance.

This complex position can involve object relations theory in a normative dilemma. If one values both the autonomy of natural society's sites and individual subjectivity's ability to search for fulfilment through independent and creative action, what happens when the two clash? Should we primarily respect the independence of sites such as homes and communities and stand back from them as much as possible, or should we be involved in the relations between the weaker and stronger participants within these sites? Object relations theory's move from libido to attachment settles this question by dissolving the polarity between its terms. Individuality's value and the necessity of social and communal sites are not mutually exclusive. The move to attachment obviates classical psychoanalysis's mooring of psychic structure in the competition for physical gratification. Consequently, society does not appear as forcing an external break with that gratification. As Guntrip (1961: 116–117) noted, even where object relations authors presented their theory as an elaboration on Freud, the move from drive to relating meant a completely different notion of the mind than Freud had offered: it meant a self that was healthily communicative and could in principle live a rewarding life within his or her community.

As understood by Ian Suttie, Fairbairn and Winnicott, attachment is not a limited resource. Interaction is its own reward, having no climax and no bottom line (Fairbairn, 1952: 79–80, 82–88; Suttie, 1999: 3–6; Winnicott, 1991: 95–100). Keeping company confiscates nothing from general usage. Attachment occurs between individuals who can recognize each other as such. It is not a merging of selves. When mothers are confident enough to gradually create distance from their young children, Ian Suttie (1999: 99–101) thinks, no anxiety infests the process: the child experiences it as continuous and does not register the trauma that would occur if a third agent, such as the father, were sensed as dramatically interfering between mother and child. If no substantial anxiety is activated, clinging is avoided, and the existence of the other person as distinct from the self can be peacefully acknowledged. Beyond the nursery, this dynamic entails that differences of perspective and interest can be tolerated and are factored into relationships, which are not expected to be total and encompassing. Any adult relationship involves a dimension of selfish exchange that satisfies each partner separately. Winnicott (1991: 86–94) formulates this insight as the ability to use the object. While sharing in social sites does not essentially impinge on the self, the self's quest for realization is not exhausted by these sites and involves the presence of an unsocialized, intensely personal ingredient that is not necessarily made available to others.

The analysts' attitude to the notion of property can illustrate the political implications of viewing attachment and social engagement as potentially synergetic rather than as conflicting with distinct and creative individuality. Suttie (1999) sees the shift from preoccupation with the mother herself to taking interest in external objects and activities as a mark of individual development (16). Undergoing this transformation broadens the individual's range of interaction. Concrete objects and activities are utilized within the process. Within it, property is a communication channel, a material basis for interaction. Overriding preoccupation with property becomes a measure of alienation from society only under conditions where the child's communication with the mother is hampered. This results either in the child's attempting to compensate by denial of dependence or, more extremely, by aggressively controlling the mother, or yet, in denial of the distance opened up from the mother. These undesired consequences are represented by the false polarity of harsh capitalism and extreme socialism. While apparently conflicting, the two positions essentially overlap by stressing the excluding, individual-centred character of property. Presented as essential for personal liberty by capitalists, the strict exclusion of others from one's belonging becomes the one character of property when castigated by socialists. Both positions register an infantile rebellion against parental neglect by denying the social and communicative aspect of property (Suttie, 1933). Winnicott (1991) similarly views property as a dialogic medium. The transitional object is the child's 'first possession' (1–2): external to the child's body, it is treated by others as continuous with the child's personality. For the child to safely retain the transitional object at as a repository of maternal attention, the environment should respect its meaning for the child and refrain from challenging the child's view of it. Having an enclosed corner from which others consent to keep away is necessary if communication between self and these same others is to develop. The notion of possession combines the imperative to respect individual entitlement with the understanding that these entitlements are valued for their social, relationship-oriented potential. Using one's rights to engage with peers is contiguous upon using one's thumb or blanket to communicate with one's mother. Rather than embattling one party against others, concepts like hallowed personal autonomy, rights and property enable individuals to interact. There is no necessary contradiction between the autonomy of internally propelled development and the integrity of social sites.

The resulting outlook retains liberalism's familiar components through a similar alignment to the one held by the reforming ideology of the twentieth century's first half. It champions the concept of individual rights and recognizes a hallowed private sphere structured around sites like the family and property, while also enabling individual creativity to exceed these sites. It resolves the tensions between Locke's and Mill's perceptions of liberty by emphasizing the role of sociability as a core motivation that both connects individuals to families and households, and provides the channel through which individuality may grow outwards, beyond the first relationships, to inform affairs at large and the institutions charged with the wider community.

From Privacy to Policy

The similarity between the social measures favoured by object relations theorists and those formulated by the philosophy of advanced liberalism should not be surprising at this stage. The policies recommended by object relations analysts follow two complementary guidelines. The first echoes the naturalist perception of the home as a universally given environment where the nourishing attention that infants require is provided. Object relations authors expressly support the integrity of the home and, all else equal, recommend that children be raised within their families even when institutions such as hospitals can do technically better work. This normative precept was the hub of the report Bowlby (1951) submitted the World Health Organization: institutions cannot grant the emotional continuity that families do. Winnicott (1991: 109) similarly argues that the 'first need…is for protection of the baby-mother and baby-parent relationship at the early stage of every boy or girl child's development'.

The second guideline derives from the theory's developmental view of individuality. Shielded privacy cultivates a benevolent and curious individuality that seeks to expand its range of contacts. The wider social world into which children grow is therefore continuous with privacy. Public life, including its civic and political capacities, is impacted by the weight individuals carry with them. Breaks in the continuum of care, separation from parents, separation of parents, perceived or real parental neglect, and external circumstances like poverty or war all disrupt the emergence of the healthy and autonomous personality. The deficit then feeds back into public life. Deprived of comforting internal objects, individuals will be motivated to regain the lost relationship by inflicting unease and pain on their surroundings. The failure of the early environment afflicts society by generating delinquency and intolerance (Bowlby, 1951: 15–45; Fairbairn, 1952: 40; Winnicott, 1986: 21–22). Consequently, the stability and cohesion of the polity presuppose individualized, friendly and tolerant citizens as well as the healthy home setting that make them possible. Where, Winnicott (1988: 152) writes, 'there is a sufficiently high proportion of mature individuals there is a state of affairs which provides the basis for… democracy'. By contrast, he warns, wherever the proportion of healthy members falls, the pathologies of the individual constituents undermine the collective and leave the stage for the totalitarian movements' promise of catering for people's starved attachment needs (Winnicott, 1986: 239–259). Governmental measures should accordingly address not just external protection for the home, but the home's internal workings. Object relations authors call for cultivating the nuclear family that composes two generations, two genders and a division of labour between homemaker and breadwinner (Bowlby, 1951: 47; Suttie, 1999: 43–44). As the source of healthy, cooperative and peaceful individuality, the family acts as an arm of the public good, both guaranteeing infants' need for safe attachment objects and performing as an agent of the public good where other such agents – social workers, therapists and analysts – cannot be present (Shapira, 2013: 17–18, 112–137). 'When parents can be used', Winnicott (1991: 19) writes, 'they can work with great economy, especially if the fact is kept in mind that there will never be enough psychotherapists to treat all those who are in need of treatment'. Combined, these measures constitute a polity that respects the autonomy of individuals and the privacy of families but intervenes when the health, education and safety of families and individuals are understood as demanding such intervention.

While extensive in its areas of operation, that regime is not perceived as intruding on privacy. It is itself an outgrowth of the same dynamics that pervade the underlying, natural units of home and nurture. The private and political spheres cannot be thought of as wholly separate: health, Fairbairn (1952: 85) writes, is a question 'of object-relationship within the social order'. If creativity is the shape that individual self-realization takes, and if it carries its healthy and open-ended sociability with it, then the import of these characters does not stop at the household's door. Instead, by populating the public world, healthy individuals ideally disseminate the patterns born of secure holding and attachment to further organizational levels. The polity becomes infused with the virtues of the private sphere. '[S]ocial provision', Winnicott (1965a: 93) suggests, 'is very much an extension of the family': it both acts as the family acts towards the child, and does so out of similar motivations. A liberal state that upholds individual rights and the sanctity of the private sphere while also extending its functions to areas like education, health, accommodation and the regulation of employment is one outcome of such thinking. It aligns with the policy proposals presented by the advanced liberals of the century's first half.

For both the expressly political philosophy of social-minded liberalism and the psychoanalytic theory developed by object relations authors, the desired institutional arrangement is based on a similar thought process. At its basis stands a perception of humans as potentially free and peacefully interacting in a condition that precedes and underlies all formal institutions. Political philosophers and psychoanalysts additionally converge in describing the dynamic of the units that inhabit this primary layer as one of sociability: the first motivation is maintaining company. In object relations theory and advanced liberal theory alike, the primary unit of natural society, the family, allows the formation of a well-differentiated, self-directing individual personality. While recognizing the basis of civilization in a universal condition, both political and psychoanalytical theories ascribe to that condition a dynamic and transformative character: if individuals are self-directing, then their actions and ideas will outrun the original sites from which they have sprung. For both social and psychological authors, the result is not necessarily a conflict between individual and society: as the underlying environment is structured by a friendly drive, the further motivations and interactions based on it are similarly pervaded. Differences provide the contents for fruitful communication rather than impel mutual destruction. Hence, a civic sphere founded on the autonomous subjectivities enabled by the underlying, natural condition takes shape. Political institutions can be safely charged with tasks that touch on the private sphere because they derive their values and rationale from that sphere, leading to the endorsement of welfare into liberalism. The state is an overparent; the institutional order it governs is an extension of the family.

References

Bellamy, R. (2003). The advent of the masses and the making of the modern theory of democracy. In Ball, T., and Bellamy, R. (eds.), *The Cambridge History of twentieth-century political thought*. Cambridge: Cambridge University Press, 70–103.

Beveridge, W. (1942). *The pillars of security*. New York: Macmillan.

Beveridge, W. (1948). *Voluntary action*. London: Allen and Unwin.

Bowlby, J. (1951). *Maternal care and mental health*. Geneva: World Health Organization.

Bowlby, J. (1973). *Separation*. London: Hogarth.

Bowlby, J. (1997). *Attachment*. London: Pimlico.

Bradley, (1979). Hegel in Britain: A brief history of British commentary and attitudes. *Heythrop Journal* 20 (2): 163–188.

Brooks, T. (2007). *Hegel's political philosophy*. Edinburgh: Edinburgh University Press.
Brunner, J. (2000). Freud and the rule of law. In Levine, M.P. (ed.), *The analytic Freud*. London: Routledge, 277–293.
Burns, C.D. (1919). *Greek ideals*. London: G. Bell and Sons.
Clarke, P.F. (1978). *Liberals and social democrats*. Cambridge: Cambridge University Press.
Collini, S. (1991). *Public moralists*. Oxford: Oxford University Press.
Dangerfield, G. (1935). *The strange death of liberal England*. New York: Harrison and Smith.
Den Otter, S. (1996). *British idealism and social explanation*. Oxford: Oxford University Press.
Eksteins, M. (1990). *The rites of spring*. New York: Anchor.
Fairbairn, W.R.D. (1952). *Psychoanalytic studies of the personality*. London: Routledge and Kegan Paul.
Fawcett, E. (2014). *Liberalism: The life of an idea*. Princeton, NJ: Princeton University Press.
Freeden, M. (1978). *The new liberalism*. Oxford: Oxford University Press.
Gerson, G. (2004). *Margins of disorder*. Albany, NY: SUNY.
Goodin, R. (1988). *Reasons for welfare*. Princeton, NJ: Princeton University Press.
Guntrip, H. (1961). *Personality structure and human interaction*. New York: International Universities Press.
Harris, J. (1993). *Private lives, public spirit*. Oxford: Oxford University Press.
Hart, B. (1910). The psychology of Freud and his school. *Journal of Mental Sciences* 56: 431–452.
Herman, A. (1997). *The idea of decline in Western history*. New York: Free Press.
Hobhouse, L.T. (1904). *Democracy and reaction*. London: Unwin.
Hobhouse, L.T. (1911). *Social evolution and political theory*. New York: Columbia University Press.
Hobhouse, L.T. (1921). *The rational good*. London: Allen Unwin.
Hobhouse, L.T. (1922). *The elements of social justice*. New York: Henry Holt and Company.
Hobhouse, L.T. (1924). *Social development*. New York: Allen Unwin.
Hobhouse, L.T. (1994). *Liberalism and other writings*. Ed. J. Meadowcroft. Cambridge: Cambridge University Press.
Hobson, J.A. (1921). *Problems of a new world*. New York: Macmillan.
Holmes, J. (1993). *John Bowlby and attachment theory*. London: Routledge.
Hughes, J.M. (2000). Fairbairn's revision of libido theory: The case of Harry Guntrip. In Grotstein, J.S., and Rinsley, D.B. (eds.), *Fairbairn and the origins of object relations*. New York: Other Press, 250–272.
Kern, S. (1983). *The culture of time and space 1880–1918*. Cambridge, MA: Harvard University Press.
Linstrum, E. (2014). The making of a translator: James Strachey and the origins of British psychoanalysis. *Journal of British Studies* 53: 685–704.
Locke, J. (1946). *The second treatise of civil government*. Oxford: Blackwell.
Manent, P. (1995). *An intellectual history of liberalism*. Princeton, NJ: Princeton University Press.
Mercier, C. (1910). Insanity as disorder of conduct. *Journal of Mental Science* 56 (234): 405–418.

Morgenthau, H.J. (1946). *Scientific man versus power politics*. Chicago, IL: University of Chicago Press.
Nicholson, P.P. (1990). *The political philosophy of the British idealists*. Cambridge: Cambridge University Press.
Nicklin, J.A. (1898). Ideals of friendship. *The Westminster Review* 149: 680–687.
Nussbaum, M. (2006). Winnicott on the surprises of the self. *The Massachusetts Review* 47 (2): 375–393.
Roazen, P. (2003). Freud and his followers. In Ball, T., and Bellamy, R. (eds.), *The Cambridge History of twentieth-century political thought*. Cambridge: Cambridge University Press, 392–411.
Ryan, A. (2012). *On politics* v. 2. New York: W.W. Norton and co.
Schuett, R. (2007). Freudian roots of political realism: The importance of Sigmund Freud to Hans J. Morgenthau's theory of international power politics. *History of the Human Sciences* 20 (4): 53–78.
Shapira, M. (2013). *The war inside*. Cambridge: Cambridge University Press.
Suttie, I.D. (1933). Is acquisitiveness an instinct? *Psyche* 13, 154–163.
Suttie, I.D. (1999). *The origins of love and hate*. New York: Free Association.
Suttie, I.D., and Suttie, J.I. (1932a). The mother: Agent or object? *British Journal of Medical Psychology* 12, 91–108.
Suttie, I.D., and Suttie, J.I. (1932b). The mother: Agent or object? Part II. *British Journal of Medical Psychology* 12, 199–233.
Sykes, A. (1997). *The rise and fall of British liberalism 1776–1988*. London: Routledge.
Tolman, C.W. (1987). The comparative psychology of Leonard T. Hobhouse: Its context and conception. *International Journal of Comparative Psychology* 1 (2): 85–96.
Trotter, W. (1908). Herd instinct and its bearing on the psychology of the civilised man. *Sociological Review* 1 (3): 227–248.
Trotter, W. (1909). Sociological applications of the psychology of the herd. *Sociological Review* 2 (1): 36–54.
Wallas, G. (1914). *The great society*. London: Macmillan.
West, R. (1986). Law, rights and other totemic illusions: Legal liberalism and Freud's theory of the rule of law. *University of Pennsylvania Law Review* 134 (4): 817–882.
Winnicott, D.W. (1965a). *The family and individual development*. London: Tavistock.
Winnicott, D.W. (1965b). *The maturational processes and the facilitating environment*. London: Hogarth.
Winnicott, D.W. (1984). *Through paediatrics to psychoanalysis*. London: Karnac.
Winnicott, D.W. (1986). *Home is where we start from*. Eds. C. Winnicott, R. Shepherd, and M. Davis. New York: Norton.
Winnicott, D.W. (1988). *Human nature*. Philadelphia, PA: Brunner/Mazel.
Winnicott, D.W. (1989). *Psycho-analytic explorations*. Eds. C. Winnicott, R. Shepherd, and M. Davis. Cambridge, MA: Harvard University Press.
Winnicott, D.W. (1991). *Playing and reality*. London: Routledge.

2 Love against Hate

Ian Suttie and Jane Suttie

Ian Dishart Suttie is often regarded as a forerunner of the British object relations school (Clarke, 2006: 169–170; Holmes, 1993: 23–24; Kirkwood, 2012: 19–33; Miller, 2007). His main written contribution precedes Fairbairn's and Winnicott's significantly. Despite his brief career, his declared hostility to Freud and his early death in 1935, the main exponents of object relations theory manifest his influence. Fairbairn's debt to him has been recently uncovered by Clarke (2011). Winnicott (1989: 575) and Bowlby (1999) both concede his stature. By insisting on the crucial role of the child-mother bond and by playing up sociability's priority as the child's organizing motivation, Ian Suttie heralds the change of emphasis that object relations theory caused within psychoanalytic thought. By, moreover, suggesting a more attentive posture by therapists that echoes the maternal function, Suttie preceded the later move towards a clinical setting that avoids a simple top-down meeting of expert and client.

By his own admission, Ian Suttie (1999) moved from an initial 'blind devotion to Freud' to a later determination to comprehensively revise psychoanalysis (220). By the 1930s, Ian Suttie's divergence with Freud was open, as noted at the time by Ernest Jones (Bacal, 1990: 17). It was multi-dimensional, having to do with theory and therapy as well as with philosophy and religion. Suttie largely avoided psychoanalytical publication platforms. Jane Suttie systematically translated works by Freud himself, as well as by Sándor Ferenczi, whom Jones considered a renegade, and by Alice Balint. This translation project provided a counter-canon to the Stracheys' 'classical' translation, through which Freud was and is known in the Anglophone world. In 1935, shortly before his death, Ian Suttie published his one comprehensive book, *The origins of love and hate*, in which his independent theory is methodically laid out as a non-Freudian form of psychoanalysis. While accepting parts of Freud's terminology and descriptive assumptions, Suttie's model inverts Freud's focus on the self-seeking and pleasure-seeking individual: instead, the individual is analyzed as invested primarily in being approved of by other people. When humans manipulate or even dominate others, the manipulation is not at bottom a means to a materialist end. It is an instrument for reassuring the manipulating and dominating actors that they are worthy of their victims' love (Suttie, 1999: 49).

This chapter first briefly discusses Ian Suttie's theoretical break with Freud and his alternative, maternal and benign, view of psychoanalysis. It then moves to discuss the normative and ideological questions that arise from Suttie's contribution, paying particular attention to the political implications embedded in the theory's description of a largely power-free and dynamic family situation.

Priests and Witches

As a military doctor in the First World War, Suttie noted that soldiers from different backgrounds reacted differently to an identical set of pressures. One's early environment and culture, then, had a significant input into functioning in later life (Heard, 1999: xxi–xxii; Suttie, 1923a). A holistic perspective was needed for examining both separate individuals and their society. Initially, Suttie viewed Viennese psychoanalysis as furnishing the missing link between mind and environment, and therefore providing the comprehensive approach he was looking for. Instead of what Suttie regarded as the tendency of earlier psychiatric thinking to reduce the mind to lists of drives and instincts, Freud proposed a set of interlocking principles that showed the response of the young child to the family situation as the determining psychic factor (Suttie, 1922, 1924b, 1923b).

But soon enough Freud began to seem insufficient. This was especially the case, Suttie thought, after Freud's development of his metapsychology in the interwar period. Instead of the earlier rigour which tied all behaviour and thought to a few, on the whole simple, principles, Freud now had to introduce the work of a mysterious and unaccountable death instinct (Suttie, 1925). Beyond needlessly compounding the theory itself, the appearance of the death instinct was scientifically insupportable, as it could have no basis in evolutionary biology: organisms strive to survive and propagate, and cannot have a collective memory of a previous phase, as Freud's assumption about the wish to die seemed to suggest (Suttie, 1924a).

The waning of Freud's appeal alone, however, was not enough for Ian Suttie to break away from him. As if to prove Thomas Kuhn's theory of knowledge, Suttie had to wander into the possibility of a completely alternative worldview for the process of abandoning Freud to be completed. Suttie could not revert to a fully biological, Darwinian worldview because, as he saw it, the cultural differences that controlled psychological attributes all occurred within the same, current evolutionary phase (Suttie, 1924c). Instead of biology, anthropology served as the platform for an alternative to Freud to spring from. Particularly, this had to do with the anthropological literature on matriarchal societies and the historiography of medieval witch-hunting (Suttie, 1999: 3–4). The twenties witnessed several attempts to compare the findings of psychoanalysis and anthropology (Gerson, 2009: 25). Immersing himself in these studies, Ian Suttie suspected that the potentialities inherent in matriarchy had been systematically overlooked in classical psychoanalysis. The defining input, according to Ian Suttie (1999: 3–4), was his realization in 1932 that Freud's negative view of society sprung from the emphasis on the oedipal situation and that this, in turn, was connected to Freud's overlooking of mothers – and to Freud's own ideological assumptions.

The point was initially elaborated in a series of articles that Ian Suttie and Jane Suttie authored together. Maternal inputs, Ian Suttie and Jane Suttie argue, are benevolent and central to later character: if this were not true, Freud would not turn to the oedipal situation in order to ground his perception of the mind as riven by conflict. Accordingly, the mother's own functioning becomes important. The more confident and independent the mother, the more significant her input is likely to be (Suttie and Suttie, 1932a, 1932b). Mothers, however, can only be fully confident when their status is assured by their societies. While imperfect, matriarchies are on the whole healthier societies. Matriarchal mothers have more sources of self-esteem than care of their children. They are occupied with household management as well as with other activities, and are therefore directly interested in their children's becoming independent early. They urge children to abandon clinging and excessive physical contact. This demand is endogenous to the relationship the child knows from birth. It is not imposed from the outside by a third partner and does not represent a reality principle that contrasts with maternal love. As maternal approval is important to the child and this approval is gained by the renunciation of clinging, that renunciation is part of an ongoing relationship and involves no subsequent essential strain. Separation and individuation are not opposed to love. They grow from the groundwork that is love (Suttie, 1932: 290–295). Experiencing pleasure and reality as continuous rather than opposed, the children of matriarchal civilization venture into a trusting relationship with their surroundings.

But like all societies, matriarchies are prone to change from within and incursion from without. When matriarchy transforms into patriarchy, not just the visible, institutional relations are challenged. The entire psychic makeup is placed under an enormous strain. Early medieval Europe, especially its Nordic and German regions, Ian Suttie (1932) thinks, was largely matriarchal prior to Christianity. The prices paid in mental health for its transit to patriarchal monotheism manifested in various ways, among which the practice of witch-hunting adopted towards the end of the middle ages was the most remarkable and telling one. The witch hunt reached its apex simultaneously with the Protestant

Reformation. The persecution of women coincided with the turn towards the stern masculine god of Protestantism (301). Suttie explains this coincidence by pointing to the relations between religion and the everyday experience of family life. In northern Europe, conversion to Christianity was achieved by political means rather than by grassroots proselytizing (289). Underneath this thin layer, the north retained its older structures. Northern society allowed women a broad scope within their families. Children experienced their mothers as strong and self-reliant (294).

On this civilization, Christianity was first imposed in its Catholic form. It was a belief system originally formulated for a patriarchy in which mothers had no standing of their own. In patriarchies, mothers are economically dependent upon males, and their children are their only source of prestige and their main company. Patriarchal mothers, then, have little incentive to repress their children's demand for close and persistent contact, as that would be giving away their one social resource. Accordingly, the first company children experience is that of a weak mother who lacks confidence and whose world is limited to the nursery. When children become aware of the father, they simultaneously become aware of a power differential. The first real authority is external to the first relationship. Reality is opposed to pleasure. The two will now always appear as opposites (Suttie, 1932: 300–301).

In patriarchy, it is the father, not the mother, who initiates the break from constant care. His desire breaks up the nursing couple. However, the child does not easily relinquish the proximity to the mother. Repression is external to the mother-child relationship. It is associated with anger and fear of vengeance rather than with a will to concur with the mother's wishes. Consequently, renunciation is never complete. It leaves traces in the shape of longing for dependency. Moreover, the striving for maternal closeness takes on the hue of the father's relation to the mother so that 'sexual wishes also attach…to the mother' (Suttie, 1932: 300). As desire is the father's prerogative, experiencing it invokes fear of retribution. Women arouse contempt when their inferior status is fully realized. It reminds the child of his early association with such unworthy authority. Subsequent social contact is coloured by frustration as it is a substitute for a more wholesome relationship, and is similarly marred by shame and anxiety. Children in such societies 'retain their infantile impulsiveness and aggressiveness, a resentment at the world, and a strong, regressive longing to shrink from it' (300). Patriarchal societies develop a cosmology of dread and guilt, centred around an arbitrary male god whose anger the believers may only hope to allay by abjection and sacrifice. Deferment of pleasure is always external, imposed and partial. Individuals do not give up anything voluntarily. They require force – physical or internalized – to keep them within bounds that make social living possible. Consequently, under patriarchy 'will arise the need for (auxiliary) religious repressions, atonements and other defences' (300).

The angst of patriarchal societies, Ian Suttie (1932) thinks, generates efforts to allay it, leading to humane reform movements. Such movements, however, may falter because they address the level of ideas and intellect rather than the deeper layer governing it, that of primary, profoundly internalized psychic experiences and the family environments in which they are acquired. Christianity itself had originally been formulated with the intention of reforming patriarchy. Addressing a civilization of male-dominated households worshipping a stern father-god, Christianity emphasized the humanely accessible, tolerant face of Christ, countering the fierceness of the Jewish god. Christianity made brotherly love a chief virtue, and so encouraged the fellowship that Judaism had sacrificed for the vertical relationship with the god. Christianity reintroduced physical immediacy into religion in the form of the Sacrament: by symbolically eating the god, the believer becomes one with him. Hence, some of the intimacy of the earliest relationship could be regained. Early Christianity offered what Judaism could not offer: soothing parental approval, fellowship on equal grounds and physical closeness not tainted by contempt (296). However, if Christianity alleviated the symptoms of patriarchal upbringing, society remained structurally patriarchal (301). This fact corrupted Christianity itself by impacting its ideas and rites. In patriarchy, physical tenderness is sexualized, and sexuality reinterpreted as domination and subjection. As communion was in danger of becoming degraded, Christianity had to present communion as 'pure' – in effect as a replication of infancy. Hence, it tended to relegate the believer to helplessness through the mysticism and miracles. Idealization of the mother figure through the increasing emphasis on Mary's immaculacy teamed up with a demeaning of real women to complete the separation of tenderness from sexuality, and of the actual world from the fantasy of seamless union arrived at only at the liturgical level. Institutionally, this development manifested itself in the celibacy of the clergy (298).

As it contracted the degrading, patriarchal worldviews characteristic of its native ground, Christianity mismatched with northern Europe. Catholicism forced the neuroses of the south on a society that had been free of them. Maternal obligations remained, but maternal standing eroded. With the dissemination of Catholic values, the contrast between practice and belief began to stand out. Mothers still psychically weaned their children according to their traditional role, but that was now resented by a society whose official value system denied women any standing. Once 'clerical anti-sexuality and anti-feminism...had weakened the actual maternal repressions characteristic of Teuto-Celtic cultures...a lively Oedipus wish and dread was awakened among the people' (Suttie, 1932: 299). Consequently, despite its original, benevolent intent, Christianity ended by destroying matriarchy. Catholicism allowed for the adoration of an ideal female figure through the cult of the Virgin, but it harmed real mothers' and women's position in society, therefore diminishing the possibility of the healthy, nearly painless weaning process that only mothers could manage in their children. The religion itself was too weak and ambivalent to contain the rage generated by its encounter with pagan society. Hatred of women erupted in collective violence, as in the persecution of witches, marking, Suttie (1932: 299–301) writes, 'the transition from Pagan-Teuton culture to Catholic and feudal culture'. To regain its equilibrium, northern Europe had to import Protestantism as an external source of repression that concurred with its new derision of women. More 'affectively akin to...Judaism' than Catholicism, Protestantism was about self-denial, guilt and shame (289–290). The craving for contact, now understood as sexual, was repressed by fear of an overwhelming external power.

Occurring simultaneously, the witch hunt and the reformation represented efforts to repress women. Their shared legacy was a self-perpetuating malignance: with their pestering guilt, shame and hate, violent patriarchies drive out peaceful matriarchies. By the twentieth century, patriarchy had become equivalent to civilized life itself. The alternative had been suppressed. In this civilization, Freud's emphasis on sexualized libido and murderous hate makes sense: 'As Freud ranks himself with the moderns, presumably he means machine guns, poison gas and bombing planes' (Suttie, 1999: 234). Freud's psychoanalytic theory perpetuates the social values it rose out of.

A Benign Alternative

If this is Ian Suttie's criticism of Freud, it is completed in its affirmative, prescriptive ramifications. To revise psychoanalytic theory and account for the healthier dynamics of matriarchy, some other factor had to fill in the place that sexuality occupied in classical psychoanalysis. Evolution, which Ian Suttie considered one of Freud's blind spots, stepped in to provide this motivation. Natural selection made humanity a primarily sociable species. Born defenceless, humans first look for others' company as it is the condition for the fulfilment of other necessities. Substituting sociability for sexuality allowed Ian Suttie (1999: 256) to finally weave the threads of his separate concerns into an 'extensive reorientation... of Psycho-analysis'. Children are born sociable but disorganized and so lacking distinction, but then, prodded by an evolutionary imperative, immediately seek contact and attention. This sequence entails that the recognition of the other person as such appears against a background that is originally devoid of differentiation and therefore instils the notion of 'all experience as unitary' (29). When the other materializes as an object of craving, alterity is not sensed as an essential break but as part of that unity: 'The love of others comes into being simultaneously *with the recognition of their existence*' (30). Individuality and community, differentiation and wholeness are therefore held together within the comprehensive framework which is the child's mind.

In the healthy and biology-based course of things, mothers foster this ability to acknowledge alterity as part of a shared, integrated experience by responding to their children's needs with tight care. Frustration is not allowed to drive a wedge between self and other: 'a true, "balanced" Symbiosis' is maintained (Suttie, 1999: 53). Inevitably, however, other demands sooner or later intervene, such as those generated by the arrival of younger siblings. However, the child's need for company is still operative. It is still focused on the mother, and it is still integrated with the holistic background of the child's experience. Psychic, as well as physical, weaning is now required. Once the child is somatically organized enough to find interests in the environment, the mother can deflect the child's attention from herself. Instead of physical contact and continuous focus on the infant, mother and child are now capable of sharing a song or a picture book. These external objects are meaningful to the child because of the mother's perceived investment in them. The child's sensation of safety no longer requires the unbroken presence of the mother herself. The focus on tangible items prepares the infrastructure for communication with others, besides the mother. Maternal attention therefore serves as a gateway for engagement with the external world. Play and conversation, music, sports and art all follow this opening: 'culture-interests...are substitutes for the...relationship of child and mother' (16). Moreover, for Suttie (1928), each individual's wish to be together with others, alongside the ability induced by maternal care in early childhood to recruit external interests into relationships, generate verbal communication, abstract thought, and therefore science and progress:

> A triangle of interest is really formed, self-other-and object, which enhances the pleasure of mental play with the idea of the object and supports that play with definite words and indicative gestures. I regard the social interest, the social situation, as the essential incentive to, and support of, the pleasurable reminiscence and fantasy reconstructions from which the function of conceptual thinking originates. (36)

While what might strike the later observer here is the way in which Suttie anticipates Winnicott's notion of transitional phenomena and their role in enabling culture and thinking, some attention has to be given to the internal makeup of Ian Suttie's work. The possibility of deflecting the child's attention towards a third, external object that stands between mother and child fleshes out the idea of endogenous repression that Ian Suttie says is the working principle of matriarchies. Mothers are capable of extending the caring relationship into new spaces that, paradoxically, require less immediate care. To do this, however, the mother requires motivation and capability. Both depend on her broader social functions, having to do with her standing and prestige. If these are lacking, the successful loosening of contact is less likely to take place. The mechanism of gradual distancing accounts for the benevolent nature of matriarchies. As it allows children to separate and individuate without lingering pain, this device makes for a more peaceful social organization. The initial nurturing experience extends to siblings, peers and the wider society. A benign circle is established. As the origin of all creative activity, sociability advances the species. Humanity constantly develops new interests and ideas that are all modified forms of communication. These innovations make for the marked progress that humanity enjoys (Suttie, 1999: 19–20).

Since a benign quest for validation and company is the primary drive, then, Suttie (1999) thinks, the incidence of confrontational behaviour points to a disturbance (125). When the child finds it difficult to tolerate the loss of the mother's constant attention, resentment builds up. The external world is perceived as intrusion and threat rather than as an occasion for engagement. The unease generated by this process manifests as illness (43–45). The individual may attempt to deny the importance of the mother – and hence of society generally – and shut himself or herself in the inaccessible universe of madness; the individual may resort to clinging and protesting his or her weakness, and so become incapable of personal independence; the individual may also attempt to gain attention by force, as seen in the preoccupation with power and material achievement; and the individual may develop a hatred of the world that manifests itself in delinquency and violence but 'owes all its meaning to a demand for love' (23).

But patriarchy trains itself not to see this truth. Where mothers are weak, they are unwilling and unable to deflect the child's primary interest away from themselves. The child's interest in external reality is not properly awakened, so that the ability to communicate with others is hampered. With the realization of the father's power, children in such societies enter a full-blown oedipal phase, in which the need for contact is sexualized and fraught with anxiety and guilt. This is the civilization described by Freud and in which his theory makes sense. Classical psychoanalysis disseminates the idea that sexuality is the repressed key to all behaviour. However, Ian Suttie (1999) points out that sexuality is not really repressed. Its direct expression is lauded in males and its indirect expression in females. The discussion of sex as the buried truth under civilization covers up something else: the loss of sociability's own legitimacy. Beyond babies, humans are not supposed to openly admit to needing each other's company. Where mothers are denigrated, early relating and the total dependency it entails are a source of embarrassment. Any sensation that takes adults back there is denied. Human interchange is therefore never left alone, for fear of the immersion in each other of the first bond. Relationships are always functionalized as commerce, debate, therapy – and sex. Modern society suffers from a 'taboo on tenderness' rather than on sex (80–96).

Ian Suttie frames the difference between his vision and the one held out by Freud as ideological. Freud normalizes the harsh, deadlocked patriarchal world in which there is no escape from conflict. Suttie himself, by contrast, is openly more optimistic and forward looking, as he knows that matriarchies existed and illustrated the possibility of a more peaceful existence. The basic need is not for competition-generating material goods, but for contact with others. Facing reality and functioning within it are not opposed to maternal love, so that no opposition between pleasure and reality needs to be assumed. Individual separation and the ability to act autonomously concur with sociability and the recognition of one's ties to others. Individual separation is continuous with love, so that no burning pain is left to poison future life (Suttie, 1999: 117–118). 'I am convinced', Ian Suttie (1932: 303) writes, '...of the possibility of an Oedipus-free culture'. By accounting for both health and pathology, by drawing on evolution and by linking individual development to the wider social pattern, sociability links up the various strands of Suttie's thought. Considered as the master drive, sociability makes sense of the place of sexuality itself as a physical sensation that gains its significance from its ability to carry an interpersonal, social load (Suttie, 1999: 72). Substituting sociability for sexuality positions Suttie fully as Freud's rival: it contrasts a hopeful vision of society with the worldview of classical psychoanalysis.

The possibility of a better world inherent in the idea of matriarchy leads Ian Suttie to an active stance towards social institutions. For Freud, remedy was private, as society was mired in perpetual struggle. For Ian Suttie, by contrast, therapy should begin where illness begins – in the environment. His own view of psychology, Suttie (1932: 303) writes, holds implications 'for mental hygiene, social harmony, and everything that concerns the cultural, "spiritual" welfare and destiny of man'. Aggression and its many manifestations – intrusion on one's fellows, attempts to seal off one's boundaries from the environment and efforts to take over others' belongings by theft, robbery and other means – are all consequences of environmental factors rather than inborn qualities. Change in the social surrounding would cultivate changes in conduct. In their co-authored article, Suttie and Suttie (1932b: 210) write that while it 'is idle to dream of a scheme of upbringing which will make smooth the path from infancy to childhood and from childhood to adult life', it is realistic to expect an arrangement that keeps 'substitution as nearly abreast with privation as possible, so that the associative impulse shall develop without serious hitch from infancy to fellowship...then mateship and finally parenthood'. Interest in such a project had to be polity-wide rather than private, because the preventative measures required for health were environmental and pertained to a much wider population than those who actually were referred to treatment or sought it actively. Freud's psychoanalysis showed the prevalence of neurosis as a hidden condition that underlies everyday function. But Suttie's revision of Freud showed that this could be avoided by addressing the surrounding conditions, thereby placing an obligation on the society to act:

> The need of the sufferers from "nervous breakdown" is great, the need of those on the way to this condition is greater, but the need of those who are able *only by wasteful effort and needless suffering* to save themselves from such disaster, is greatest of all by reason of the much greater numbers in this latter situation.
>
> (Suttie, 1929: 83)

In operative terms, Suttie thought that such understanding meant broadening health services, primarily by placing more clinics at the general public's reach.

In clinical terms, Ian Suttie's theoretical shift entailed that therapists should acknowledge the illness usually arises from a deficit of love and seek to remedy this illness at its root. Among the rest, Suttie warns, this means that the passive, blank-screen analyst upheld by classical analysis should be abandoned. Such a standoffish posture is in itself a sediment of both the Freudian preoccupation with power and domination, and a practical perpetuation of the power relations which Freud thinks pervade all relationships. Ideally, Suttie (1999: 251) writes, the analytic setting should establish 'a rapport with the physician in which the patient can have the utmost confidence; and under cover of this new-found confidence the true work of "reduction" may be commenced, namely *the reduction of grievances*'.

Ian Suttie does not elaborate on the institutional settlements his approach may involve. What he does say points in the direction of a welfare mechanism. The complexity of industrial society makes it difficult to fully reclaim matriarchy. The demands of the workplace necessitate full-time engagement, and so make child-bearers dependent on breadwinners. However, pressures on mothers may be significantly minimized and their status enhanced by measures that would bolster their ability to initiate healthy weaning. Mothers' capability to see their children through a relatively painless process of separation rests on the special position of the mother in the home. For Ian Suttie (1935), their inability to occupy that position indicts wage-earning mothers or mothers who experience their children as a burden as psychically and socially harmful. Society may help by protecting the mother-child relationship from the poverty that makes mothers severely dependent on others or otherwise sends them to seek employment outside the home. Once assistance is offered and families are geared to rearing healthier children, such symptoms are expected to decline.

Exclusion and Conformity

Despite the optimistic and liberating resonance of Ian Suttie's outlook, it includes some troubling elements. Particularly, Suttie grades cultures normatively. Matriarchies provide the conditions for benevolent repression. Their beliefs and organization reflect the healthy approach that individuals take when their fundamental sociability is not warped by anxiety and aggression. Patriarchies, by contrast, foster submissive mothers, dominating fathers, weak and untidy forms of repression, and hence resentment and aggression – and the ideological tenets to justify them. The opposites of health and illness roughly correspond to the Nordic and Mediterranean regions. In the north, matriarchal 'Pagan Teutondom' was characterized by 'the highest imaginable practical standard of conduct' (Suttie, 1932: 290, 292). The pathology of the south – what Suttie and Suttie (1932b: 218) call its 'faulty, unbiological system' – gradually took over and destroyed northern matriarchy. When Catholicism, already corrupted by centuries of Mediterranean influences, intruded on the north's harmony, it introduced '[g]reed, violence and superstition, alternating with a regressive flight from the world' (Suttie, 1932: 300). In its initial attempt to heal patriarchy, Christianity introduced 'the conception of social life as based upon Love rather than upon authority' (Suttie, 1999: 140–141). Whatever eventually went wrong with Christianity was a result of its encounter with the culture which it tried to reform: 'the Christian tradition has been transmitted through emotionally distorted minds' (146). Catholicism developed the features that it later imposed on pagan matriarchy, thus leading to the further complications of witch phobia and Protestantism, which Suttie perceives as a reformulation of Judaism, the religion of southern patriarchy. From solution, Christianity declined into a problem. Southern patriarchy was the culprit in this process.

Ian Suttie (1999) frames his own contribution as a move in the grand arch of this intercultural war. He points out that psychoanalytic practice began from a pre-theoretical stage in which the therapeutic powers of interpersonal communication were given free scope. In the 1880s, Joseph Breuer's talking cure had pointed to its own explanatory theory: love and recognition heal the patient. While later denied by Freud, this intuition was retained by him in practice, and was given some theoretical body by Sándor Ferenczi (203–217). But in its classical, full-blown form, Freudian theory replicates the hatred and envy of patriarchal society. As his theory pits pleasure against reality and individual against society, Freud perpetuated the governing pathology. Instead of showing patients the possibility of love, Freud composed a 'childish hymn of hate' (255). Being a distortion of an earlier sound intuition, Suttie concludes, 'Freudian theory is itself a disease' (218). As such, it aligns with other social diseases, such as totalitarianism and war, whose reliance on naked force overlaps with Freud's perception of hate as constitutive. 'One is almost inclined', Ian Suttie wrote in the early 1930s, while the Berlin Psychoanalytic Institute was being shuttered by the Nazis, 'to assume that Freud is among the prophets who will be quoted by those exclaim "Heil Hitler"' (234). The process by which the talking cure became metapsychology shares its pattern and its main agents with the process by which Christianity became Protestantism. Like Christianity, psychoanalysis was eroded by contact with patriarchy – and a specific patriarchy at that. 'Freud's own antecedents', Ian Suttie writes, 'lie in perhaps the most patriarchal of all cultures, a circumstance which, along with his preoccupation with the neuroses, led him to discover the paternal repression first' (104–105). Judaism's 'sense of guilty apprehension' poisoned both ancient and modern attempts at regaining mental health (196). The north-south, Teutonic-Jewish divide that distinguishes matriarchy from patriarchy, therefore, is operative not only in the history of religion. It also manifests in the history of psychoanalysis, implicating Freud and positioning Suttie himself as the herald of a new psychology that would be free of the cultural trappings of classical psychoanalysis.

These remarks and their implications have drawn attention and criticism (Gerson, 2009; Zaretsky, 1998: 35). The critical tone is perhaps best seen in the work of Hewitt (2018), who raises the concern that Ian Suttie's work diminishes Jews by casting what Suttie thinks is their culture as particularly harmful, while placing an idealized version of Christianity, now shorn of any Jewish connections, as the benevolent alternative. As Ian Suttie has been lionized by later psychoanalytic and broader scholarship for initiating the move towards a relationship-based psychoanalysis, it becomes that scholarship's burden to extricate object relations theory from its supremacist origins:

> Even more unsettling is that Suttie is writing in the historical context of 1930s Europe, portraying Jesus as inaugurating an ontologically superior, 'Nordic' Christianity against an inferior 'Semitic' Judaism. Contemporary scholars of Suttie must acknowledge that his ideas are hopelessly compromised by racist-inflected fantasies that constitute an inextricable part of his criticisms of Freud. It then becomes possible to see the disturbing parallels between a Christian anti-Judaism based on a historically inaccurate and untenable understanding of 'early Christianity as a completely new religion', and an object relations theory that breaks with Freud by introducing a 'new' psychology [of] love.
> (237)

If later object relations theorists do not sufficiently address this issue, Hewitt (2018: 235) asks, are they not complicit with Ian Suttie's bigotry? If these inheritors of Suttie's work accepted his constitutive ideas without denouncing the additional baggage that in Suttie's own work seems inseparable from these ideas, do they not endorse that baggage too? Some evidence exists that can provide an indicting affirmative answer. The independent group of British psychoanalysts, in which object relations ideas were dominant and in which object relations theorists were prominent, formed in the space between the feuding camps of Anna Freud and Melanie Klein, both German-speaking and Jewish immigrants. Doane and Hodges (1992: 30) point out that Winnicott's occasionally rosy description of motherhood and the family came from the heart of a traditionally male-dominated, Christian and native-British middle-class consensus. Other researchers describe how the ethnic, cultural and class prejudices that haunted the middle group sometimes made it to the surface through backroom remarks (Rodman, 2003: 403). A part of Ian Suttie's appeal to these analysts may have had to do with what Suttie upheld – and with what he berated and excluded.

Here, another troubling aspect of Ian Suttie's approach becomes synergetic with his ethnocentrism. It is his approval of conformity and his dislike of pronounced waywardness. For Suttie, the ability to participate in one's culture is a mark of health, while excessive criticism of one's environment raises the suspicion of occult resentment towards one's mother. A patient Ian Suttie (1924d: 618) saw manifested his illness by showing 'no feeling for the delicacies and niceties of social intercourse'. By contrast to such symptoms of illness, conformity at this level becomes a testament of health. Accordingly, for Suttie (1999), therapy should be seen as 'a reconciliation of the patient to his social and cultural environment' (248). If Freud wanted to teach patients to accept the irreparable rift between themselves and the world – the inaccessibility of total gratification, the divisive role of sexuality and the unacknowledged hostility towards one's parents – then Ian Suttie's idea of clinical work points in the opposite direction. He would rather convince patients of society's benevolence. The therapist assures the patient 'that there can be nothing in his own mind wholly alien to the mind of the analyst, or alien to...the other patient from whom the analyst has learned'. Consequently, 'the patient comes to realize that there is no intrinsic difference between himself and anybody else' (251). The outcome of such therapy is that the wish to draw away from society, challenge it or assert one's distance from it all dissipate, along with the psychic pain to which they give rise: the anger and alienation initially sensed are themselves pleas for love, which the analyst's tolerance guarantees. 'The patient', Suttie writes,

> then dares to face and admit his anti-social impulses, regressive and aggressive; he voices his age-old challenge to the mother's love, and in so doing discovers that the social separation-anxiety to which it gave rise is in reality quite uncalled-for, since he was really loved and since his *protest* is kindly received.
>
> (251)

Social connections, the motivation and feeling of reward gained by maintaining them, and the sense of living in familiar environment are all essential for health, and admitting the need for them is the basis for health. By way of translating this insight into broader principles, Suttie proposes 'the maximum amount of tradition and continuity' and 'the minimum prejudice to the adaptability of the social structure' (121).

Suttie contrasts this conventionalist attitude with Freud's deliberately oppositional approach: the issue is not just matriarchy against patriarchy or north against south, but also the familiar and reassuring against the alien. For Suttie, Freud's hateful attitude manifested itself in iconoclasm. Freud's psychoanalysis deliberately contravened the norms and conventions of its time in the name of scientific rigour. Suttie (1999) offers his own work as an attempt to save psychoanalysis' useful therapy from its counter-intuitive and asocial metaphysics. The abstract, detached posture of science, which Freud imports into the clinical scene in the shape of the largely silent analyst, 'is an antithesis to the Christian religion which seeks to reconstitute the tender relationship...which is lost in early childhood' (3). Suttie's theory and the compassionate therapy it entails are organized to 're-introduce common-sense into the science of psychology': an effort to purge psychoanalysis in the same way that early Christianity purged monotheism of its guilt-ridden elements (259). Suttie provides an ideology and a militant voice to the turn that the practice at the 'parson's clinic' took away from classical psychoanalysis. He pits optimism against gloom; social engagement against seclusion; compassion against aloofness; pure-hearted Christianity against Judaism; North against South.

This equation of the familiar with the morally good fits a broader pattern than just the psychoanalytical milieu. As accounted in the previous chapter, British liberal reformers cultivated the notion of the loving home as a national symbol that contrasted with what they saw as Europe's stress on internal discipline and external conflict. That symbol and the way of life associated with it were seen as coming under threat during the first decades of the twentieth century, not just because of the consequences of poverty and war, but because of the scepticism and nihilism that emanated from the Continent, as in the vitalist philosophy of Nietzsche and the morally neutral posture of functionalist sociology. To this was added an influx of imported art forms and aesthetic fashions, a phenomenon felt especially after the First World War. These trends all amplified a diffuse apprehension of cultural siege and an overall sense of dislocation, in which desire and aggression subverted trust, love and normality. It was an atmosphere in which it was possible to question and even ridicule convention in everyday life, as well as in art and politics. Freudian psychoanalysis, with its emphasis on sexual desire as a multiform and ever-present motivation, was understood as one of these disruptive elements (Gerson, 2004: 13–18).

Ian Suttie (1999) shares the local dislike of these importations, casting Freud as a private case of the larger pattern. Much of what the period saw as innovation in thought and art, Suttie thinks, were forms of the taboo on tenderness, replacing as they did the older intellectual, literary and artistic venues whose values were intuitively accessible to all: 'it seems possible that refuge from tender feeling and pathos generally is being sought in sex and that this flight is expressed in some people's intolerance of "good" music and delight in jazz excitement' (85). By contrast, Suttie's alternative psychology anchored the theory of mind to the more familiar landscape of household and fellowship, casting itself as defending a threatened civilization against an external threat. Contemporary responses to Suttie's work approved of his ability to bring the reassuringly familiar back into psychology. One anonymous reviewer (1936) lauded Suttie for refuting the opinion that 'has found…its crudest expression in such a statement as "Every mother is her child's first seductress" – an opinion so monstrous as to prove of itself that its originator is incapable of understanding what maternal love means'. An overall attachment to intuitively accessible values, among which the nuclear family and an idealized form of motherhood were central, features to varying degrees in midcentury object relations theory. Jeremy Holmes (1993: 215) characterizes Bowlby's work as reaching back through Freud to a more stable Victorian world. The British school's theory may consequently be thought of as a local, nationally based reaction against the unsettling impact of Viennese psychoanalysis and the wider intellectual alliances attributed to it. The cultural, ethnic and regional aspects that Suttie cites in his opposition to Freud accord with the implicit assumptions and priorities of the other analysts and of a wider section within the educated public. Suttie's conventionalism and ethnocentrism are not wholly alien to these analysts: these features may be blatant and exaggerated representations of their own perceptions.

However, there are also mitigating circumstances that can be shown to lessen the burden of the analysts' alleged complicity with the ethnocentrism Ian Suttie manifests. Suttie's principled disagreement with Judaism as a religion does not necessarily spill into a rejection of Jews as humans. Suttie does not case his ethnocentrism in essentialist and deterministic terms. Professionally and ideologically, Suttie aligns himself with Breuer and Ferenczi, who were as Jewish as Freud, without showing any sign of discomfort: the biological, deterministic category of race, a ubiquitous issue in the 1930s, was clearly not at stake for him. And if other object relations authors shared Ian Suttie's aspiration towards a new psychology that would rescue the received, insular, Victorian and particularly Christian world, they did not necessarily endorse Suttie's equation of Christianity or humanism with a geographical culture or a national identity. Fairbairn is often compared with Suttie because of their Scottish background and religious humanism (Bondi, 2013; Clarke, 2006: 137–149;

Miller, 2008). Fairbairn, however, values Christianity because it installs a sense of discipline and differentiation, accustoming its adherents with a complex, never perfect world, rather than offering them the unconditional maternal embrace of Suttie's version. For Fairbairn, demanding from faith such an unconditionally rewarding approach was itself pathological. An overly intense identification with any religion and its god figures is as indicative of illness as is unreserved attachment to the state that terminates the ability to criticize it: both are regressions to an undifferentiated, infantile phase. Fairbairn thus disagrees with Suttie's emphasis on communion and the offer of immediate closeness as the defining, beneficial characters of Christianity. Moreover, Fairbairn clearly does not share Suttie's Nordic, pre-Christian affiliation. Fairbairn (1952) identified German National-Socialist ideology with 'the old pagan Teutonic culture', which he contrasted with 'the traditional Classico-Christian culture of Western Europe' (252). If object relations theory follows Ian Suttie, it follows Fairbairn too: the journey departs from normative ports that are close in many ways, but cannot be condensed into each other. While the later analysts did not denounce Ian Suttie's remarks on ethnicity, they could clearly hold a different perception than his on these matters.

Whatever the final balance on the implied nationalist and ethnic contents of object relations theory, Hewitt's criticism of Ian Suttie points to another source of rigidity in his work: the pitch of its social optimism. While shunning downright utopia, Suttie offers a vision that involves a nearly perfect accommodation of society to nature and of each individual self to the other. As such a sweeping resolution of social and individual angst is in principle available, contesting it has to be an attack on nature and the prospects of human happiness. The horizon for a legitimate non-utopian social criticism diminishes. Such a pre-emption is a central ideological motivation for Suttie's elaboration of an alternative psychoanalysis. Freud had a critical edge: his theory is sceptical about any certainty or comfort. It is necessarily disruptive, and involves, as Hewitt (2018: 227) writes, 'an uncompromising examination of those "dark" parts of our intellectual traditions, and our entanglement with them, that thwart our efforts toward bringing about the "right kind of society"'. Suttie opposes Freud on this very point: Freud does not just err methodologically. He derails society's advance by stressing the prices and discontents involved in social life.

It is essential for Ian Suttie that these discontents are not determined by biology or any other natural or universal factor. They are in principle avoidable. By allowing for a process of relatively painless growth into adulthood, Suttie suggests a social meliorism based on natural forces and natural groupings such as the family. It links individual health to the social environment within a framework of principles that apply to all social sites, from the cradle on: sociability and love are primary and natural, while aggression, hatred and resentment are secondary and distorted. Discontent can be addressed by care and by environmentally aiding the mother to provide care. On the basis of this framework, a normative and policy agenda for the entire civilization becomes feasible. The 'central task of mankind', Suttie (1999: 125) writes,

> has been maturation and the harmonization of his love-needs with his appetite needs and the attainment of maximal satisfaction in both. It is a task which must be pursued simultaneously in the developing, adapting, *individual*, and in the ever-changing *community*.

As this potential alignment of individual happiness with social good is anchored in a fundamental truth about humans, it cannot be legitimately opposed: such opposition perpetuates the sickness by normalizing it. For Suttie (1999), Freud's account of humans as violent animals ends in accepting 'conquest as evidence of superiority' (227). This casting of people as hostile and aggressive by default stems from an initial refusal to concede the constitutive character of love and recognition (231). Denying the fact of primary, underlying sociability generates an 'attitude to life [that] is of necessity correlated with a pessimism and aggressive attitude which…we find in all Freud's writings' (232). Addressing the sickness as if it is anything but sickness is immoral, as it blinds us to the possibility of correction. Freud's disruptive, unsettling stance is disqualified because it is disruptive and unsettling. What Suttie's theory excludes is not just a specific group: it is the availability of a social criticism that does not take the possibility of harmony as its departure point.

Matriarchy and Politics

Ian Suttie, then, makes it difficult to debate issues in terms of differing interests and the conflict that can arise out of them. For him, it can be said, where quarrel, and therefore politics, were, harmony, morality, and psychological knowledge will be. Nowhere do the results of this approach show more consistently than in his perception of gender. Suttie frames gender as an essential and biologically determined division of tasks. Maintaining that division is conducive to the peaceful social order he has in mind. The unit based on the reproductive and caring mother on the one hand, and the breadwinning father, on the other hand, is not a subject for enquiries that proceed from the assumption of conflicting interests.

This can be surprising, because Suttie sides with women's demands for equality and recognition. His work anticipates the feminist perspectives of Benjamin (1988) and Chodorow (1978), as it places Oedipus and its strains within the context of the patriarchal household, and proposes that mothers be understood as full, autonomous and rational agents.

Along with Jane Suttie, he understands the status of women as not just a question of justice and equality for them alone, but also as crucial to the entire social order's health. The mother provides the child with the first instance of another subject like the self who is both relatable and independent: from here, the later ability to communicate with peers and tolerate their differences follows (Suttie and Suttie, 1932b: 220, 228). Resolving gender through the empowerment of mothers thus has a beneficent impact on all social relations.

But the feminist thought that developed since the intervention of de Beauvoir (1989) also involves the realization that individuals' aspirations and interests cannot be subsumed under those of other individuals and cannot be papered away by reference to biological necessity, genuinely felt emotion or a transparently natural order of things. Feminist thought usually shuns appeals to a pre-political natural state or a post-political end state. In the absence of constant challenge and critique, sexual differences reify into power differentials that are placed beyond debate because they seem natural rather than political (MacKinnon, 1989; Okin, 1989). Ian Suttie's worldview contrasts with this feminist emphasis on the pervasiveness of politics. When Suttie substitutes sociability for libido, Freud's warlike world transforms into a more hospitable place. Evolution endows infants with an ability to detect response in others. Unless disrupted, a mutually respecting relationship between self and other is built from the first hours of life on. Society begins with nurture. Beyond this foundation, the availability of endogenous repression entails that essential conflict need not arise. 'There is', Suttie (1999: 39) writes, 'no abiding sense of insecurity or of grievance'. The mother has a similarly benign perspective on the relationship. 'Still less', Suttie (38) writes, 'is it possible for the child to offend the mother; all its acts are absolutely acceptable; it is both "free" and "good"'. Under social arrangements that give significant standing to motherhood, people may retain this experience and extend it to other interactions.

The viability of an overall conflict-free civilization is based on a gendered family setting where women are the primary care-givers. That setting is grounded in biology. Evolution, Ian Suttie (1928) thinks, favours individual variability within a species as a survival strategy, as it makes for a greater pool of skills. In humans, cooperation puts these skills at the service of the collective, rendering the combination of variability and cooperation especially attuned to evolution. The simultaneous growth of individuality and cooperation is reflected in the development of the human family unit, where each adult is treated as a separate and unique individual – rather than as an interchangeable member of the horde – and where each is given a specific role: man or wife. Individuality is therefore not opposed to sexual specialization, but is instead related to it through evolution (Suttie and Suttie, 1932a: 104–105). Specialization in parenting tasks is accordingly a central feature of human adaptation. In lower life forms, Suttie and Suttie (1932b) argue, fathers share the direct care of the young, but in the more complex species, the 'higher evolution of the reproductive function…tends to leave the male out of the family in an effective and physiological sense' (212). Hence, the emergence of the ambulatory male is a consequence of a biological process rather than a product of social bargaining. This process allows the 'further specialization of the female for the nurture of the young', thus helping women to fulfil themselves (213).

The internally structured family is therefore a natural, essentially conflict-free phenomenon in which the welfare of the entire society is grounded. As consequences of human evolution, gender roles are placed beyond political enquiry. Women should be content and proud when performing their single, preordained function. The natural process that led to the creation of the healthy family leads women away from any public role. Women, Ian Suttie (1999: 117–118) writes, '"drop out" of society' because 'family life affords to them a more complete satisfaction of the social need'. Applying to women a mechanically egalitarian rationale meant to enable them to act as men is inimical to women's own good as it ignores their distinct, gendered function. Jane Suttie (1922) warns that applying the terms of juristic equality that dominate public life to the home dangerously counters biology. Pondering what she understands as women's vulnerability to psychiatric symptoms, Jane Suttie attributes it to modernity's preoccupation with disembodied, abstract egalitarianism. Owing to it, economic and political agency are made the measure of everyone's worth. Twentieth-century women are accordingly pressured to perform not only their traditional tasks, but also the competitive ones historically reserved for men. 'Women', she warns, 'are suffering from a growing deviation of interest from biological objectives' (550). Consecutively, women find themselves crushed by contradictory obligations. The stress endangers not just women as individuals, but the entire society, as it hinders the vital, parental role that women play. The accumulating pressures are potentially apocalyptic: 'civilization after civilization has waxed to some such height of female emancipation as we enjoy to-day and then collapsed' (551). While the social order should respect women so as to enable them to function as mothers, that respect differs from the entitlements usually associated with constitutional democracy. Instead, Suttie and Suttie (1932a: 96) assert, women deserve conditions in which to develop their 'self-esteem as women'.

The question now arises of what Ian Suttie means when he uses the word 'matriarchy' as denoting a historical model of a healthy society. In its dictionary sense, 'matriarchy' is a political order, a government by women. If matriarchal women are predominantly mothers and mothers should not be understood through vocabularies taken from the realm of publicity and politics, what does the word 'matriarchy' as used by Suttie denote? Suttie describes the pagan north as matriarchal. In that society, women and motherhood were respected, and children grew up into an adulthood that was not blemished by envy. While notoriously violent in their dealings with the world outside, the Scandinavians were internally peaceful because of the operation of endogenous repression. Women took care of everyday life, while men were away at sea. Women could in these circumstances take on traditionally masculine roles in their closest ambience (Suttie, 1932: 294). Nonetheless, women would never take men's place at sea or war. For matriarchy to carry on, they had to devote their lives to child rearing. Any attempt to change this settlement represents an effort by men to usurp women's place. Envious of the females' reproductive and nurturing capacities, men might have tried to take on the parenting role for which they were 'functionally unfitted' (Suttie, 1999: 122). Men, it seems, carried the instruments of coercion and exploited the possibilities gained by their being exempted from household care. Were men, then, not really the rulers in this environment, which should therefore more accurately be described as patriarchy?

Aware of this possible question, Ian Suttie replies that 'matriarchy' does not denote a political order. Suttie (1999) assesses that women cannot actually rule a whole society as a matriarchy. Too many adjustments would have to be made for them to do so. Among these adjustments one may expect a neglect of maternal duties, which scuttles that civilization's entire rationale: 'a truly matriarchal *society* is an abnormality...which hardly, if ever, can exist' (120). Accordingly, the term should be understood as denoting the family structure and little else:

> When I talk of matriarchy, I mean a state of society where the woman is the effective head of the household so far as the young children are concerned, and where, consequently, the matriarchal family organization affects the character and maturity of the adults as well as, to some extent (a less important matter), the formal structure of society. (120)

So long as mothers appear authoritative to children, their other functions, rights and status components feature as instruments to their function. Women's subjective experience – their own thoughts about their position and manifold ways of responding to the challenges involved in it, the possibilities they give up to men so as to be able to loom large in the children's world – all these have become secondary.

Suttie's vision, then, depends on a fundamental depoliticization of the home and its permanent organization along the lines of unequal division of tasks. This outcome follows on Suttie's overall dislike of considering issues of conflicting interests: the natural, biology-based society he envisages pre-empts essential envy and aggression, leaving the observer with no political or juristic instrument with which to gauge the home's own workings. Even raising such questions betrays the Freudian, pathological involvement of patriarchal thought. Suttie propounds a view in which much of our existence is negotiable, as we can be made largely free of neurosis. At the same time, as Zaretsky (2015: 105–106) notes, Suttie also believes in certain unnegotiable essentials such as the biological grounding of parenting roles; the same essentialism reverberates in his attitude to cultures and ethnicities. As conforming with these essentials is also presented as natural, healthy and moral, then diverging from them, questioning them or suggesting that they are the outcomes of power structures are all condemned as sick and immoral.

Conclusion

Ian Suttie's achievement is impressive in many ways. While being largely shunned by orthodox analysts, he, along with Jane Suttie, authored a wholly new form of psychoanalysis. While endorsing the conversational therapeutic method from Freud, Suttie installs that method within a different theoretical model. At its core stands not Freudian libido, but the need to relate, attested to by the intuitively recognizable dependence of infant on mother. Societal and cultural conditions impact the relationship between child and mother. In its healthy mode, society enables the mother to be confident enough to gradually wean the child from the immediate, unceasing care that biology demands in the first months of life. When such a distancing has been achieved through the mother's own agency, it is absorbed by the child as part of the relationship rather than as a threat to that relationship. This makes for an individual constitution that calmly accepts the fact of dependence but is able to move beyond it to full adult autonomy. But societal conditioning can go wrong. When the environment interferes with maternal agency, healthy growth cannot be completed. Weaning from direct attention is experienced as a consequence of an external disruption and is associated with the father's image. Individuals growing up with weakened mothers are distressed by their own dependence, a condition which leads them to deny it and emphasize emotional distance, domination and exploitation. A culture arises in which quarrels, conflicts, emotional apathy and the denigration of women are regarded as normal. Hobbes, and in psychoanalytical theory, Freud, write from within this ailing culture and mistake its distortion for reality. In this way, Ian Suttie and Jane Suttie construct the ideational and normative platform for later object relations work, placing the need to relate at its centre, and establishing the environmental responsibility for the rise of individual autonomy that links the psychoanalytical thought of midcentury Britain to contemporary progressive and liberal approaches to politics.

At the same time, the theory Ian Suttie promotes extracts some normative prices. Visible primarily in the theory's gradation of cultures and therefore inviting questions about its ethnocentric assumptions, Suttie's liabilities also include embellishing traditional gender roles by depicting them as natural. While upholding the significance of women to psychoanalytical theory as well as to the social good, Ian Suttie, along with Jane Suttie ground that significance in the performance of social tasks distributed by reproductive functions. Women are appreciated as physiological females acting as such, because acting this way coheres with a natural process for which the later imposition of artificial, purely formal equality is a distortion. Politics, in the sense of an area marked by relations that are determined by nothing but relative power, is part of that distortion, as the natural order is made wholly benevolent and power-free through the mother's functioning. Worldviews, such as those held by Hobbes or Freud, that place power and indeterminacy first, manifest that distortion. From Suttie's perspective they stand denounced, not just as errors but as moral travesties. Religions and philosophies that broadcast a pessimistic worldview in which struggle is inevitable betray their basis in the guilt incurred within a patriarchal culture by one's inevitable, natural need for tender response. From such perspectives, the 'world appears evil', while 'the whole attitude to life becomes ascetic and...misanthropic' (Suttie, 1999: 151). Nature, then, enables a social order that, being potentially harmonious, has no need for political or juristic terminologies. The politics of governmental enforcement, impersonal law and formal equality is associated with a disruption to that harmony. The apparently bigoted and gender-essentialist ingredients in Suttie's position are related, as both stem from an assumption about a pristine, pastoral order.

Ian Suttie's work largely bypasses Klein, as he began developing his ideas prior to Klein's intervention and mostly ignores her. The mother, for Suttie, is primarily a person not an object, a condition which serves as the groundwork for the child's growth into a trusting, and therefore genuinely independent, adult. If Fairbairn and Winnicott endorsed some insights from Klein, their attribution of neurosis to a disruption of maternal care rather than to unavoidable psychic features is more closely related to Ian Suttie. However, later object relations theorists rarely went as far as Suttie had gone in confronting Freud explicitly or in suggesting that orthodox psychoanalysis expresses a malevolent ideology. Fairbairn and Winnicott are, additionally, more guarded in suggesting the possibility of social improvement. With the assistance of Klein's model, these later psychoanalysts view the mind as underlined by ambiguity and confusion that cannot be entirely dispensed with. Their affiliation with Suttie means that they suggest ways in which maternal function can ease and utilize that ambiguity. Their level of social optimism differs. Fairbairn, especially, is reserved about the venues for translating the first relationship into a platform for a peaceful social order. This will be discussed in the next chapter.

References

Anon. (1936). Review of *The origins of love and hate*. *Journal of Neurology and Psychopathology* 16: 377.

Bacal, H.A. (1990). Ian Suttie. In Bacal, H.A., and Newman, K.M. (eds.), *Theories of object relations: Bridges to self psychology*. New York: Columbia University Press, 17–27.

Beauvoir, S. de (1989). *The second sex*. New York: Vintage.

Benjamin, J. (1988). *The bonds of love*. New York: Pantheon.

Bondi, L. (2013). Between Christianity and secularity: Counselling and psychotherapy provision in Scotland. *Social and Cultural Geography* 14 (6): 668–688.

Bowlby, J. (1999). Foreword. In Suttie, I.D. (ed.), *The origins of love and hate*. London: Free Association, xv–xviii.

Chodorow, N. (1978). *The reproduction of mothering*. Berkeley: University of California Press.

Clarke, G.S. (2006). *Personal relations theory*. London: Routledge.

Clarke, G.S. (2011). Suttie's influence on Fairbairn's object Relations theory. *Journal of the American Psychoanalytic Society* 59 (5): 939–959.

Doane, J., and Hodges, D. (1992). *From Klein to Kristeva*. Ann Arbor: University of Michigan Press.

Gerson, G. (2004). *Margins of disorder*. Albany: SUNY.

Gerson, G. (2009). Culture and ideology in Ian Suttie's theory of mind. *History of Psychology* 12 (1): 19–40.

Heard, D. (1999). Introduction. In Suttie, I.D. (ed.), *The origins of love and hate*. London: Free Association, xix–xl.

Hewitt, M.A. (2018). Christian anti-Judaism and early object relations theory. *Critical Research in Religion* 6 (3): 226–242.

Holmes, J. (1993). *John Bowlby and attachment theory*. London: Routledge.

Kirkwood, C. (2012). *The person in relation perspective*. Rotterdam: Sense Publishers.

MacKinnon, C. (1989). *Toward a feminist theory of the state*. Cambridge, MA: Harvard University Press.

Miller, G. (2007). A wall of ideas: The 'taboo on tenderness' in theory and culture. *New Literary History* 38: 667–681.

Miller, G. (2008). Scottish psychoanalysis: A rational religion. *Journal of the History of Behavioural Science* 44: 38–58.

Okin, S.M. (1989). *Justice, gender, and the family*. New York: Basic.

Rodman, F.R. (2003). *Winnicott: Life and work*. Cambridge, MA: Perseus.

Suttie, I.D. (1922). Critique of the theory of 'Herd instinct'. *Journal of Mental Science* 68: 245–254.

Suttie, I.D. (1923a). Some aspects of sociology and their psychiatrical application. Part I. *Journal of Mental Science* 69: 49–51.

Suttie, I.D. (1923b). Some aspects of sociology and their psychiatrical application. Part III. *Journal of Mental Science* 69: 314–318.

Suttie, I.D. (1924a). Metapsychology and biology. *Journal of Neurology and Psychopathology* 5: 61–70.

Suttie, I.D. (1924b). Moral imbecility. *Journal of Mental Science* 70: 362–363.

Suttie, I.D. (1924c). The development and evolution of mind: Biological versus psychological interpretations of the ontophylogenetic parallelism. *Journal of Neurology and Psychopathology* 5 (18): 133–145.

Suttie, I.D. (1924d). Two cases illustrating the conception of moral imbecility. *Journal of Mental Science* 70: 612–626.
Suttie, I.D. (1925). An unwarranted accretion to the Freudian theory. *British Journal of Medical Psychology* 5: 83–91.
Suttie, I.D. (1928). The evolution of social thought. *Psyche* 33: 31–36.
Suttie, I.D. (1929). Psychotherapeutic clinics. *Psyche* 37: 82–84.
Suttie, I.D. (1932). Religion: Racial character and mental and social health. *British Journal of Medical Psychology* 12: 289–314.
Suttie, I.D. (1935). Mental factors in the welfare of the child. *Public Health* 48: 294–301.
Suttie, I.D. (1999). *The origins of love and hate.* London: Free Association.
Suttie, I.D., and Suttie, J.I. (1932a). The mother: Agent or object? *British Journal of Medical Psychology* 12: 91–108.
Suttie, I.D., and Suttie, J.I. (1932b). The mother: Agent or object? Part II. *British Journal of Medical Psychology* 12: 199–233.
Suttie, J.I. (1922) Mental stresses of adjustment in women. *British Medical Journal* 3221 (23): 549–551.
Winnicott, D.W. (1989). *Psycho-analytical explorations.* Cambridge, MA: Harvard University Press.
Zaretsky, E. (1998). Melanie Klein and the emergence of modern personal life. In Stonebridge, L., and Phillips, J. (eds.), *Reading Melanie Klein.* New York: Routledge, 33–48.
Zaretsky, E. (2015). *Political Freud.* New York: Columbia University Press.

3 Ronald Fairbairn and the Legacy of Prussian Idealism

Ronald Fairbairn, the 1889-born, Edinburgh-based psychiatrist and analyst, defined the very concept of a psychoanalysis that is rooted in relating to an object rather than in satisfying a physical drive (Kernberg, 2000; Mitchell, 2000). Seeing patients privately in the 1930s, Fairbairn (1952: 84–85) noted that many of them do not respond well to interventions based on the classical Freudian model. Fairbairn accordingly proposed a shift of focus from a self who seeks gratification to one who seeks relationship with an object. Taking in parental inputs, the child organizes his or her psychic structures to accommodate the wish to relate to the object on the one hand, and the object's own perceived character and acceptance of the child, on the other hand. Psychotherapy and psychological theory should, Fairbairn concluded, address these modes of object seeking and object perceptions as their fundamental material (82). As Clarke (2011) shows, Fairbairn was influenced by Suttie's views. In his turn, Fairbairn was acknowledged by Winnicott as an inspiration (Levy, 2014: 246). Like Suttie, Fairbairn was interested in retrieving a comprehensive, holistic and humanist approach to society from the clutches of a potentially reductive method of enquiry. Science, Fairbairn (1952) argues, should not make us lose sight of the moral concerns and ethical choices involved in social life. Presenting phenomena such as crime, deviance and distress as narrowly medical subjects springs from a regrettable 'general modern tendency to substitute purely scientific standards for the moral standards of the past' (290–291). This, he warns, 'represents an interpretation based upon an erroneous psychopathology' (291). As in Suttie, therefore, Fairbairn's turn from sensory gratification to a preponderant sociability was partly motivated by a normative, even ideological concern. This orientation will later reappear in Winnicott.

To an extent, Fairbairn appears to share the liberal, progressive and welfare-oriented positions of the other analysts. Fairbairn upheld democracy as a political ideal, and sought to configure it in ways that reflected the findings of psychoanalytic theory. The social order had to accommodate the object-seeking mind (Fairbairn, 1952: 85). Government could be understood both as a remote extension of the home and as an aid for the home's functioning. An effort to provide the needs of homes and families, alongside political democracy, were the instrument for shouldering this task.

Like other psychologists, Fairbairn was active within the nascent web of state services. He was a consultant to the Ministry of Pensions, a governmental organ tasked with administering the safety-net insurance payments that became the hallmarks of the Beveridge Plan. In thought and action, then, Fairbairn manifests the overall alliance between British psychoanalysis and the rise of the distributive polity.

However, there are elements in Fairbairn's perspective that stand out from the other object relations authors. More cautious and less intuitive in style than Ian Suttie and Winnicott, he was also aligned philosophically with the perceptions of mind and society suggested by Hegel in the early nineteenth century (Birtles, 2002, 2005). Hegel was a constant, if ambivalent, presence in British social thought: his holistic approach to individual and collective life was attractive enough for reformers striving to counter the ascription of overly individualist and hedonic motivations to humans. But Hegel's valorization of the state's power and his strict perception of social hierarchies and exclusions also placed him under a cloud of suspicion for liberals. The affiliation with Hegel accordingly makes for a position on politics and citizenship that somewhat distances Fairbairn from the other analysts.

To discuss this position, I first outline Fairbairn's theory, and then devote a section to the relevant fundamentals of Hegel's thought and to his reception by British social thinkers. I next point to Hegel's overall proximity to the object relations stance, and then focus on Fairbairn's perceptions of the state's interface with the family, citizenship and the legitimacy of political exclusion. Fairbairn's developing ideas and the shifts of emphasis within his work have been described by Kernberg (2002), Mitchell (2000) and Scharff (2005). His historical and textual links to likeminded psychologists, as well as his intellectual roots in social Christianity and in the Scottish enlightenment have similarly been uncovered (Clarke, 2006; Miller, 2008; Sharpe, 2016). I largely take these complexities for granted. I examine Fairbairn's work as a single oeuvre.

From Drive to Relationship: A Genealogy

Unlike Ian Suttie, Fairbairn was not openly confrontational towards Freud. Instead, he presented his modification of classical analysis as a necessary development that follows on elaborating the internal logic of psychoanalysis itself. The turn to an object-relating subject, Fairbairn (1952) writes, was already incipient in the way that Freud and Karl Abraham envisaged libido as a determining force that moves through the human organism. Freud and Abraham, however, unnecessarily focused on the various erotogenic zones impacted by that force as if they were its authors:

> The historical importance of the libido theory and the extent to which it has contributed to the advance of psychoanalytical knowledge

> requires no elaboration; and the merit of the theory has been proved by its heuristic value alone. Nevertheless, it would appear as if the point had now been reached at which, in the interests of progress, the classic libido theory would have to be transformed into *a theory of development based essentially upon object-relationships.* The great limitation of the present libido theory as an explanatory system resides in the fact that it confers the status of libidinal attitudes upon various manifestations which turn out to be merely *techniques for regulating the object-relationships of the ego.* The libido theory is based, of course, upon the conception of erotogenic zones. It must be recognized, however, that in the first instance erotogenic zones are simply channels through which libido flows, and that a zone only becomes erotogenic when libido flows through it. *The ultimate goal of libido is the object;* and in its search for the object libido is determined by similar laws to those which determine the flow of electrical energy, i.e. it seeks the path of least resistance. The erotogenic zone should, therefore, be regarded simply as a path of least resistance; and its actual erotogenicity may be likened to the magnetic field established by the flow of an electrical current.
>
> (31)

The creation of an object relations approach is therefore both declared a pioneering innovation and reassuringly placed within the bounds of the psychoanalytic family as one of its organic members.

Fairbairn accounts for it, moreover, as a particle of genealogical sequence in which Melanie Klein stepped in to cover Freud's theoretical deficits and was later herself modified so as to smooth out an internal inconsistency in her perception. Some patients appeared to Fairbairn (1952: 84–85) inaccessible to Freudian intervention: while they spent a considerable time in treatment and were attentive to the analyst's interpretations, they showed no improvement. The oedipal sediment has been excavated, but something else lurked beneath. Klein provided a clue as to what that could be, as she focused on the first phase of life, a period earlier than the oedipal stage. If going there could unlock some patients, Fairbairn concluded, then it could account for most of the others as well: the early, mother-dominated stage of life was the widest common denominator. Accordingly, Fairbairn (168–175) endorsed Klein's description of the mother's role in enabling the child's integration from initially disorganized somatic and psychic components.

However, in a move that will become a constant feature of the object relations approach, Fairbairn dispenses with Klein's reliance on inborn aggression (Grotstein, 2000). Again, the move seems derived from intra-theoretical concerns. Klein entails that the initial paranoid layer of the personality grounded in the child's original disorganization is never fully transcended and that, moreover, people differ in their abilities to develop the second, social and so-called depressive layer. The fragility of this second layer is common, which accounts for the efficacy of the method based on Klein's theory. But that commonality itself required a reconsideration of the theory. Illnesses based on the paranoid position manifest in adults who are mostly functioning rather than in delusional psychotics, as one would expect them to be if the infant was a bundle of terror and hate. Another factor, then, has to exist to counteract the various destructive forces from the very first stages of life. Fairbairn (1952) suggests that this factor is the wish to relate. A profound confirmation of the self is gained for the child by relating to an object, usually the mother (72–73). If the object is perceived by the child as neglecting or as overstimulating, the need to relate to it does not disappear. It partly transfers to internal objects that take on the rejecting and overstimulating features of the original object, while a central portion of the self still interfaces with that original object (59–70). Psychic forms of organization, including healthy and neurotic patterns, all follow on this internal relationship: all of us live in a world governed by the initial responses of the society around us to our need for attention and closeness (Clarke, 2006: 24–25).

Hence, instead of a struggle between inborne drives, some of which are intensely destructive, one was looking at an internalized model of how the very young child senses the surrounding society, along with the child's own place within that society. This perception served as the groundwork for other object relations theorists. As it stood on the shoulders of Freud and Klein, this new perspective was not presented as some wild innovation, as in Ian Suttie's framing of his own work, but as a product of a cooperative dialogue between different generations of analysts. Summing up Fairbairn's significance for the development of the theory, Guntrip commended it for finally letting go of the cognitive hindrances that held back the culmination of psychoanalytic thought. If, by framing the concept of the super-ego as an internalized father image, Freud had introduced the possibility of understanding the mind as an internal conversation, he had been too constricted by his reliance on physiology to fully admit its social, dialogical, character. Freud accordingly kept falling back on instinctual explanations that burdened his perception. By contrast, Fairbairn allowed the combination of Freud and Klein to transform psychoanalysis itself:

> The elaboration in *Great Britain* of a different theoretical orientation… developed the concepts of *the 'internal object' and the 'inner psychic world' as parallel to external objects and the outer world*; and so comes to correlate the internal and the external object-relationships in which the personality is involved. This development arises out of the work of Melanie Klein and others and is worked out in a systematic and comprehensive way by Fairbairn.
>
> (Guntrip, 1961: 51).

But despite Fairbairn's playing this foundational role, his endorsement of Hegel's ontology comes between him and the other object relations authors. That ontology, along with some of its ideological elaborations, is outlined immediately below.

Dialectic and Society

Hegel views reality as mediated through the mind. Essentially unified, the mind always divides against itself, as it grasps every concept partially, which invites the discomfort generated by the presence of the parts not grasped. As additional inputs are constantly met with, discomfort with the aspects of these inputs that the mind has to neglect accumulates to a breaking point. This results in the reorganization of perception to accommodate both the previously processed and the previously neglected particles. But as perception is always partial, the new organization soon encounters its own blind spots, precipitating another crisis. These 'enlightened' and 'dark' sides of human perception are referred to as thesis and antithesis. Their dynamic of conflict and reconciliation is known as dialectic. Every element in Hegel's model derives its meaning from its place in the dialectic phase in which it appears: what is objective, final and exhaustive now may become subjective, partial and provisional later, when sufficiently troubling new inputs are met with and the mind has to relegate all its contents to new roles. All social processes at all levels of organization replicate the dialectic pattern. Wishing to engage with others in order to receive validation, we invoke in those whom we meet a reply that, as it emanates from another mind, questions our own received perceptions. If we are to be rewarded by these others' validation, we should pay by validating them, or else relegate them to the status of mute objects which cannot validate us. For a rewarding confirmation of our worth, we burden our own certainties with those generated by others. As others are similarly motivated, they, too, are transformed by the interaction (Brooks, 2007).

As the world is perceived through the mind and the mind is structured by dialectic, knowledge and society are similarly structured. The social institutions we live in embody a currently feasible arrangement of past theses and antitheses. These institutions nonetheless accrue an antithetic pressure that is indecipherable to our cognition, as that cognition is a constituent of the current phase. Based on this perception, Hegel (1952) recommends that individuals be geared to the fullest participation in their current social system, which incorporates previous theses and antitheses, thus furnishing the highest level of integration and the fullest realization of the self available at that point in time. As it contains all these ingredients, society is multilevelled. Its units range from the smallest and most physically intuitive – the family – to the broadest and ethically most fulfilling – the state, a collective that has a legitimate monopoly on lethal force. The state's harshness is testimony to its significance. Citizens would kill and die for it, thus making the state more than a contractual relationship where individuals seek to maximize gains. The state is the site where people acknowledge, through risk and death, that they are obliged to the world around them. The apparently contradictory demands that the intimacy of the family and the impersonality of state make on the citizen should be arbitrated by placing them in a hierarchy. Hegel uses the eponymous character of Antigone in Sophocles' play as an illustrative device. Having attempted to assert the demands of kinship by burying her renegade brother in contravention of governmental edict, Antigone is buried alive. Neither denied nor elevated, kinship lies subdued beneath the more advanced structures of politics and law (Beaney, 2009; Honig, 2013: 192–193).

Hegel's outlook seems to be at odds with the main trajectory of Anglophone liberal philosophy. This has two main aspects. The first is psychological. Locke and the utilitarians shared the notion of the mind as malleable and impacted by the impartation of specific facts, rewards, pressures and the chain of associations that they trigger. These thinkers favoured education and debate as engines of improvement. As debate depends on its specific participants and their particular environment, progress is gradual and uneven. Social systems should reflect this by showing tolerance and limiting their own scope. Hence, an incremental and rationalist approach to knowledge attaches to these variations of liberal thought. Hegel, by contrast, sees conflict as the engine of progress. We learn by encountering resistance: thesis can only morph into synthesis after colliding with the antithesis. Debate, rational persuasion and verbal discussion have little to do with this process. Conflict and sacrifice are inescapable features of human fulfilment, establishing the force-wielding sovereign as the last instance, diminishing the value of democracy and perpetuating war. If we follow Hegel here, we should think in wholes rather than in fragments and increments. Minds, civilizations, historical phases and knowledge systems are all interlocking within and mostly impervious to substantial input from without. Cataclysmic upheaval alone changes them. As long as such upheaval has not occurred, there is no point in comprehensive reform or deliberate reorganization (Bradley, 1979; Franco, 1997).

Despite these mismatches with constitutional liberalism, some late Victorian and Edwardian social authors in Britain found Hegel's thought valuable. He seemed to address a lacuna in liberal theory itself. The naturalist and utilitarian bases of liberal thought were minimalist. Stressing individual liberty, they were reluctant to discuss collective goals for society or prescribe desired conduct to individuals. Liberal theories defined legal and illegal, legitimate and illegitimate, free and unfree, but they did not always provide answers to what was ethically or spiritually desirable. Hegelian idealism, by contrast, delivered a comprehensive view of mind, society and history that linked all aspects of our shared existence to each other. While respecting individuals as such because all those social aspects had to be channelled through their minds, Hegelian philosophy showed that the primary good that society gave individuals was validation and the opportunity to be meaningfully valuable to others. As the good of every individual entailed living in a society and society was ideally geared for a collective existence that considered each of its particles, society should be understood as more than the sum of private interests. Hegel could consequently be helpful for late Victorian and Edwardian social reformers interested in cultivating solidarity and mutual responsibility. These authors and activists endorsed Hegelian inputs in various ways and formulations (Den Otter, 1996; Morrow, 1984; Nicholson, 1990).

For some early twentieth-century liberal thinkers, incorporating Hegel also meant that liberalism itself had to be modified. If individuals could be fulfilled only within a social framework, then a commitment to discipline and possibly risk and sacrifice had to be considered as a part and parcel of individual liberty. Consistent Hegelians like Bernard Bosanquet (2001) equated personal fulfilment with visible participation in society as it currently stands. Its fundamental unit is the family. While the couple are attracted sexually, sexuality derives its significance from 'a need for union, and an attraction outside the immediate self' (101). The family has itself to be acknowledged by the external world. It generates objects for the world to see, such as offspring and property. Preoccupation with these objects urges breadwinners on, despite hardship. The household's significance renders it a subject of special recognition by the state (171, 187). Bosanquet similarly affirmed the state's own significance as the synthesis of all other associations. Those who concentrate on 'exclusive objects', such as the family or the church, are 'prey to stagnation' (103). While patriotism might appear to conflict with attachment to one's family, allegiance to one's country is a commitment to what binds together all households and is a validation of our social, other-oriented nature (176).

For Bosanquet (1910), the same set of considerations also meant that welfare services should be offered by government, but that these services should nonetheless be limited. The issue of employment has to do primarily with acting on a genuine motivation to contribute and sacrifice, not with economic circumstances and material reward. The same can be said for spending, economizing and setting an order of priority for the family: people have to desire deferring gratifications and withstanding difficulties as manifestations of their commitment. Advice may be offered to the needy so as to give them means with which to productively tackle their difficulties, but they are expected to strive on their own. People who lack the will to make good use of this counsel and seek direct relief instead exclude themselves from full citizenship. The population is accordingly split in two – the citizens and the intentional paupers, who are placed beyond the pale of participation. This outlook remains within the scope of liberalism because it leaves its main institutional features, such as elections and constitutions, in place, and, more substantially, because it allows the individual full discretion over his or her life. If one is excluded from civic life, that exclusion is a reversible choice made by that individual.

These efforts to combine Hegel and liberalism met with criticism for their potential of straying from egalitarian norms, causing a certain backlash among social thinkers. It was aggravated by the First World War. The conflict brought with it a general dislike, shared by some intellectuals, of ideas that were identified with Prussian and German nationalism. Hegel was among the targets. Against this background, Fairbairn can be read as siding with the liberal and democratic interpretation of Hegel's thought. This affiliation is asserted through psychology rather than directly through social philosophy.

Hegel and Object Relations

On its own and in its original, Freudian, variant, psychoanalysis is not compatible with Hegel's idealism. Based on the permutation of a physical drive and its frustration by the external world, Viennese psychology was individualist and materialist. It focused on what perceived scarcity does to a personality organized around its corporeal needs, thereby aligning itself with the view of the mind as distinct from the world, opposed to it and malleable by it, as in Locke and Mill. In Britain, the liberal reformers of the early twentieth century could be sympathetic to psychoanalysis because it placed some of the responsibility for individual well-being on the material, economic, environment, grounding demands for tackling poverty and economic uncertainty. At the same time, however, orthodox psychoanalysis bolstered a rigidly individualist, even capitalist, view of humans as pursuing material ends and little more. A turn to a more sociable, holistic view of the personality could therefore furnish a plausible route for socially sensitive psychologists and other social reformers to take. But that required a change in psychoanalysis itself, one that would allow for both the individualist component proposed by Freud and the communal perspective illustrated by Hegel.

As detailed by later relational theorists such as Benjamin (1999) and Ogden (1992), much of the object relations worldview is suffused with Hegelian notions. For Hegel, the self constantly seeks validation of its wholeness and realness. It finds that validation in love. The elevating experience of love stands for our intuitive acceptance of our own relativity. For a certain moment, genuine devotion to another person incorporates our previously apprehended realization of our not being totally independent, without destroying our sense of self in the process.

This concept of validation through committing social bonding may shore up a more potentially optimistic outlook than is allowed by Freud. We are driven, not towards some uneasy compromise between our desires and an alien world that constantly withholds satisfaction, but towards a more integrated existence that connects us to others. Whether or not expressly deriving from Hegel, this insight underlies the revision of Freudian theory by object relations theory. People are made who they are by relating, and relationships are dynamic, moving from one contradiction or paradox to the next, with objectivity and subjectivity changing places rather than representing fixed positions. The infantile illusion of omnipotence and parental compliance with it give rise to mature recognition of dependence, while at the same time and on a different plain the infant is dependent and the adult gives sustenance. Maturity neither disowns the childlike fantasy of omnipotence nor seeks to fulfil it. Adult personality is a synthesis that incorporates earliest holding as well as its loss.

These parallels between Hegelian and object relations thought work well on the individual level. They strain, however, when reaching generalization about society and its ends. In Hegelian thought, the state and its use of force are essential. Dialectic tension is resolved on each social level by deferring it to the next, until the ultimate level of organization is reached and conflict becomes an unavoidable feature. In the object relations literature this is not necessarily the case: conflict need not erupt, and acknowledging its reality by showing willingness to risk and sacrifice is not the measure of the healthy mind. For Ian Suttie, as we have seen, appropriate maternal care has the power to delete any traces of the frustration its gradual withdrawal causes. Where the mother is confident enough, she is capable of gently distancing herself from the child by turning the child's attention to shared pursuits. She is freed from the need to cater minutely. Children do not grow up with pent-up anger. In a society based on such families, aggression is marginal. By contrast, aggression becomes widespread in cultures that cast women as inferior, and where, as a result, mothers find it difficult to wean their children from direct care. In such cultures, children view the mother as both weak and frustrating. The result is that any deep bond is a source of shame, as it points back to dependence on a feeble woman. Despising tenderness, such a society would put a premium on aggression (Suttie, 1999: 78–79, 93–96, 101–105). Suttie's world therefore divides between wholly good and wholly bad options for the organization of society. On its one side, he places a peaceful matriarchy where mothers are strong and adults both self-confident and capable of caring relationships. On its other side, he places a warlike society of aggressive males and subjugated females, with both genders tormented by the sediments of infantile dependence. Cycles are either benevolent or malevolent, and the contact between the good and the bad cycles contaminates the good and destroys it.

Similarly, for Winnicott (1991), health depends on a sense of creativity, which, in turn, hinges on the infant's realization that one can share an interest with the mother instead of focusing on her directly. This opens up possibilities of shared pursuits that can extend from the peer group to the rest of society. Making a difference to the world by staking out one's psychic contents in shared, transitional space, one grows out of illusory omnipotence, connects to others and develops a sense of autonomy. One is therefore expectant rather than suspicious about others' differences from one's self. In health, the dynamic of attachment is basically identical within the family and outside it. Care transcends any specific location: it extends from the home to culture while enfolding and minimizing the import of institutions charged with enforcement and collective defence. However, when the process fails, the individual perceives life as futile, and would therefore resent the creativity of others. From this derives a need to limit and dominate others, which 'eventually could build up into a dictatorship' (Winnicott, 1986: 232). Such pathologies may arise from disruptions such as war, in which families are separated and homes broken. This outlook, in which cycles are not dialectic but are instead either benevolent or malevolent, distances Winnicott and Suttie from the social notions espoused by Hegel, for whom conflict at some level is unavoidable and for whom the personality is measured by its ability to participate in the force-wielding state which is valued precisely because of its difference from the home.

Wholes and Splits

Hegelian insights thus appear only intermittently in most object relations literature. They rarely extend from the individual to the societal plane. But Fairbairn, to whom several of the object relations strands can be traced, stands out against this background. His affiliation with Hegel is consistent and systemic. It informs his clinical and social perceptions alike, distancing him from the worldviews of Ian Suttie or Winnicott.

Hegel's prevalence for Fairbairn's worldview can be glimpsed in Fairbairn's presentation method. Despite ascribing critical significance to infant life, Fairbairn rarely describes childcare in detail. Uniquely among contemporary male analysts, Fairbairn was an active parent who cared directly for his own children (Fairbairn, 1987: 21–22). This may go some way towards accounting for his avoidance of such idealizing passages about parenting as occasionally characterize Ian Suttie and Winnicott, but it makes the paucity of nursery concretization in his work even more outstanding. His treatment of what happens in early life has a technical ring to it. It proceeds along formal axes of splits and phases that he presents in diagrammatic form. One reason for this may be that such axes and splits are, for Fairbairn, largely independent from context: the shapes they take are local variants of a universal structure. When conceptualizing that structure, one may legitimately overlook local detail. With Hegel, Fairbairn views the mind as essentially unified, but at the same time as universally divided. As Grotstein (2000) writes, Fairbairn insists on the initial wholeness and innocence of the child's personality. This initial wholeness echoes Hegel's perception of the mind as ultimately unified. But its fragmentation is, as in Hegel's perception of a dialectic struggle, equally global. The coexistence of unity and division manifests in the map Fairbairn (1952) draws of the variegated internal objects and the self-parts relegated to engage with them. The self's internal division is practically universal, as some frustration within the nursing context is unavoidable. This division corresponds to Klein's paranoid position. At the same time, being essentially unified, the mind holds out a horizon of integration. The early division, then, may be gradually transcended by the more mature capability to interact with external reality and real others, a development which corresponds to Klein's depressive position (82–151).

The depth of Fairbairn's commitment to the view of mind as simultaneously unified and divided may also be illustrated by considering the notion of what Fairbairn calls the exciting object and its corresponding libidinal self. Why should excitement, in the sense Fairbairn ascribes to it, generate a split? Libido, for Fairbairn, is not a proto-sexual physical drive as it is for Freud, but the quest for an object. Perceived neglect or censure on the parent's part is experienced by the child as acute distress that results in internal restructuring. However, excitement is a surplus not a deficit of relating: it is 'overdoing a good thing' (Scharff, 2005: 8). What in such an experience of the object invites a crisis which is equivalent to the frustration of the ego's drive towards relationship while actually deriving from the undue satisfaction of that drive? Possibly, the answer is that the object's presence challenges the self's original unity. Maternal attention might overwhelm the system with inputs from an otherwise valued source. Unlike the introjection that follows rejection by the object, this distress does not derive from a threat to the self's value. It derives from a threat to the self's structure: to its internal contiguity. The self organizes against this threat by relegating the task of meeting it to a specialized portion. Original wholeness has therefore to occupy an axiomatic status within the model similar to ego's being relation-seeking. Fairbairn has to assume an original and therefore essentially integrated whole, for which excitement is a threat. Universal wholeness, however, is immediately succeeded by equally universal division. 'This would not hold true', Fairbairn (1952) explains, '…in the case of a theoretically perfect person…but then there is really nobody who enjoys such a happy lot' (8). Both the original integrity of the subject and its splintering are given. What Fairbairn describes is not a plot or a journey, but the essential condition of the psyche.

The global nature of splitting and the personality organization based on it distinguish Fairbairn from Ian Suttie. In Suttie (1999: 29), the child begins from a solipsistic illusion in which self is not distinct from the objects around it. This is transformed by the experience of the mother's relative distance. The potential frustration that follows is alleviated by proper maternal response. There is no corresponding experience of over-stimulation, unless the relationship is pathological, as happens when the mother is weak and clings to the child for her own self-esteem. Under favourable circumstances, the gradual loosening of holding is the single axis of development. Its ample management paves the road for a personality which is at once autonomous and caring. There is no question of disintegration from original wholeness, and there is no issue with the reintegration of split parts. When pathological reaction to excitement does appear, it manifests in the personality's content rather than in its structure, and its occurrence depends on local culture rather than on the universal architecture of the self. This disparity between Suttie and Fairbairn has implications for their attitude to the possibility of social perfectibility. In Suttie, infantile solipsism is replaced by healthy relating to the mother, and then to society. As repression leaves no traces, it makes possible a non-violent civilization. Fairbairn, by contrast, views ego-splitting as universal. Accordingly, he cannot envisage a culture that does not extract emotional prices. Human life is always incomplete.

Hence, rather than being a state of untarnished bliss, health is, for Fairbairn, the maximal level of integration that can realistically be achieved. It shows in the individual's ability to advance beyond the preoccupation with internal objects and their corresponding part egos without denying their existence (Ogden, 2010). Health, then, manifests as engagement with real-life objects: as the ability to gear the entire personality towards the encounter with imperfect other people in the various fora available for interaction with them. By contrast, illness is defined by succumbing to the pull of internal objects. 'My life', Fairbairn (1994) quotes a patient, 'is interfering with my neurosis' (91). Fairbairn comments that this attests to a 'tendency on the part of the individual to keep his aggression localized within the confines of the inner world as a closed system' (92). The analytic project is one in which life takes precedence over neurosis. The mature ability to concede one's emotional dependence on others while acting independently is an always-incomplete process of integration from internal constituents. It reflects Hegel's view of dialectic as the procession of mind through the incorporation of antithesis and thesis into synthesis. Fairbairn's perception similarly mirrors Hegel's social outlook, in which engagement with one's society as it now stands is the measure of the integrated mind.

Family and Polity

Before addressing some of the details involved, I should note that Fairbairn is mostly open about the stern and socially conservative hue of the worldview he acquires from Hegel. As our minds are governed by dialectic and therefore fail to process inputs that clash with the current thesis, we always live within a system of received, traditional knowledge. We cannot profoundly challenge it, and pretences to mounting such challenges might undermine society itself:

> it is safe to assume that the cohesion of every group is bound up with some ideology or other, however inexplicitly this may be formulated and however tolerantly it may be maintained. It seems inevitable, therefore, that some limit should always be imposed upon free enquiry by any social group which seeks to survive.
>
> (Fairbairn, 1952: 253)

While minds are impacted by the wish to engage with others, healthy engagement is not just an open space for creativity and personal expression. As in Hegel, meaningful engagement takes specific routes and unfolds in known locations. For Fairbairn, the family home and the national society are the two irreducible organizational levels. People react primarily to their internal balances rather than to material circumstances (Fairbairn, 1952: 234). Units based on psychological essence survive radical upheavals. The family is such a unit. It furnishes the first arena where the self's response to society plays out and consequently shapes the self. Our personalities evolve around an internalized model of how we process the first society we participated in. On the interior of our minds, we always live within family households, where we relate to attachment figures. This remains true under all circumstances, including the potential replacement of biologically based homes with more professional and managerial forms of communal caring, as in such dystopian fiction as Aldous Huxley's *Brave New World*: even then, Fairbairn (1952) predicts, 'the baby...will require to be brought up by others; and those who perform the parental function will inevitably acquire the significance of parent-figures in the child's mind' (244). Citing Freud and contemporary anthropological literature, Fairbairn writes that the family is the 'foundation upon which the higher forms of social organization and culture rest' (236). Associations based on the extension of family ties to a larger scale, such as the clan, may disappear as history moves on, but the family itself cannot disappear. Primary care is internalized in each person's mind. For all its flaws, the home is indispensable. Libido seeks an object rather than climactic gratification, and the home provides the setting for this quest. The household-based 'bourgeoisie' discipline, though occasionally constricting, is a reasonable settlement that allows infants to grow. Accordingly, Fairbairn rejects Marxism as an unrealistic attempt to resolve the internal division involved in early nurture by replacing the family with a communist collective (242). The fact that this cannot really be done, Fairbairn points out, is revealed by the Soviet leadership cult: a regime that declared the cessation of family attachments could not survive unless it presented itself as a type of family, with a father-figure at its head (244).

While the home provides the first social space and thereby furnishes the potential for the emergence of relating but autonomous individuality, that potential is fully realized elsewhere. For Fairbairn (1952: 34), mature dependence means that individuals are able to relate to each other through sharing activities that do not centre on any of them as a particular person: they engage not in, but with each other. Maturity 'involves an abandonment of relationships based upon primary identification in favour of relationships with differentiated objects' (42). The move cannot be completed in the home setting or in organizational units that extend it, as they all contain certain degrees of attention to the other as a particular person. It requires a space for impersonal obligation, and for exertion and sacrifice that distances each person from their emotional depth and focuses them on the shared effort. Civic life and the state are the site for this achievement. The national society and the territorial state it organizes into are the one permanent counterpart to the family (237–238): while the family home enables one to depend and grow out of dependence, the state allows one to fulfil maturity by acting outside specific attachment.

As both are essential, the family and the state have to coexist:

> The survival of the family as a social institution shows that the nation has failed to eradicate the family group as it eradicated the clan and the tribe, and has been compelled to make terms with the family by incorporating it into the national organization.
>
> (Fairbairn, 1952: 238)

All people find it difficult to leave their internal world behind. Consequently, the society based on healthily differentiated individuals has to contend with a constant traction back from public obligation into the more intimate experience of the household. Antigone remains a perpetual rival of the civic order as well as its necessary constituent. Fairbairn warns that 'an intense conflict still persists between the family and the state. The extent of this conflict is liable to be obscured by the fact that it is so largely a hidden or, more strictly speaking, *repressed* conflict' (238).

The polarity of family and state surfaces in crises such as war, when the ability to commit oneself impersonally demands what might be experienced as pressure to compartmentalize away one's internal world. Such conditions expose the fragility of the loyalty to the civic collective. Citizens might subsequently withdraw their attachment from society as a whole and fall back on the world of the family, with its patterns of close holding. In their minds, the home is favourably contrasted with the coldness of the organizational units beyond it. The tendency towards such regression is particularly strong in democracies, as their impersonal constitutional structures exclude the autocratic practice of presenting the leader as a relatable parent figure to whom one can emotionally gravitate when plied away from everyday life. 'Separation-anxiety', Fairbairn (1952) anticipates, 'must obviously resent a special problem for democracies in time of war; for under a democratic regime the dependent individual can find no substitute for his accustomed objects under military conditions' (80). This antipathy towards the demands of the civic public sphere, Fairbairn (1952: 281) writes, is popularly referred to as the decline of morale. It was evident in Britain during the interwar period. When totalitarian apologists mentioned the 'degeneracy of the democracies', they pointed to a real occurrence, a 'lack of public spirit', which 'manifested itself in an obvious reluctance on the part of the individual to make personal sacrifices in the interests of the national group' and in a corresponding emphasis on 'personal...and familial interests' (283).

Regardless of these difficulties, Fairbairn (1952) trusts democracy. For all its faults, the constitutional, rights-respecting polity allows for the coexistence of privacy and publicity and thus corresponds to the healthy mind's internal organization. By contrast, tyrannies elide the distinction and therefore sooner or later fall prey to the pathologies involved in the inability to ease primary attachment's hold. While totalitarian regimes seem better mobilized, this appearance is achieved at the price of turning the state itself into an early attachment figure. Citizens are not allowed to hold loyalties that differ from the collective will, which is tellingly presented to them as a close family member, usually a father character. In terms of individual health, dictatorships are badly flawed, because they do not provide their subjects with locations that can draw them out of their internally split world and offer them the remedial experience of detached, issue-focused interaction. This spells dictatorship's demise. If the state is not a truly civic and political bond, but is instead a personal one, it is subject to the dynamics of personal attachments. Frustration with politics is experienced as internal strife. With defeat or other misfortune, 'the regime becomes a bad object to the individual; and the socially disintegrating effects of separation-anxiety...assert themselves at the critical moment' (80). Citizens of democracies can at such times find comfort in their private world. The internal world of totalitarian subjects, however, is suffused with figures that have to do with the state that denies them this sanctuary. The undoing of dictatorship therefore involves worse distress than the difficulties experienced by democracies (284–285).

As opposed to the utopian horizon opened up by Ian Suttie through his perception of nearly price-free maternal weaning, Fairbairn's expectation of universal splitting means that democracy is not exempt from friction and war. Nor is democracy destroyed by war, as Suttie's matriarchy is destroyed by patriarchy. In Fairbairn, health is by definition an ability to tolerate the tensions between dependence and assertion that are endemic to the human condition, rendering democracy reasonably resilient because of its avoidance of reducing privacy and politics to each other. War may actually bring out democracy's inner strength, as it proves people's ability to add an impersonal commitment on to their primary attachments without burdening that commitment with the emotional intensity of the object world: 'in a democracy the individual is less dependent upon the state, and, therefore, less subject to disillusionment regarding the "goodness" of the state as an object' (Fairbairn, 1952: 80). Personal health, as defined by the ability to handle relationships on various levels, is validated rather than negated by the discontents of democratic life. Democracy reflects a multilevelled individual personality that can acknowledge its internal divisions without being overwhelmed by them. Attachment to both home and the sovereign collective of citizens is essential. If Ian Suttie rejected communist utopia because of what he judged as that ideology's infantile and regressive wish to do away with all differences, then Fairbairn (243) criticizes communism for its internationalism: communism does not offer a realistic political forum that can take the place of the territorial, democratic state.

Exclusion and Boundaries

Divergence from this structure interferes with individual health as it mars the individual's ability to participate as a citizen. Fairbairn suggests that such divergences be registered as milder or harder exclusions from citizenship. Such divergences, Fairbairn thinks, emerge particularly during crises such as war. Analytically inspired military doctors such as W.H.R. Rivers had used Freud as a basis for advocating a more lenient treatment for shell-shocked troops during the First World War, arguing for a conversational rather than disciplinary treatment. Commenting on similar phenomena during the Second World War, Fairbairn (1952: 285) does not preclude such a therapeutic perspective, but loads it with a more disciplinarian charge derived from his Hegelian perception of the state as the ultimate site of participation. If the horizon of the reasonably healthy and integrated mind consists of social functioning, which includes functioning within impersonal and demanding environments, then the medical expert becomes ideally an enabler of such functioning. Such functioning takes into account the call for effort and risk issued by the entire society, especially during war. Therapists should acknowledge that their mandate involves enabling their patients to participate in the collective emergency:

> Many psychiatrists who have been concerned in the treatment of the so-called 'war neuroses' have approached the problem of treating members of the services from the customary standpoint of a medical man practising in civilian life, i.e. they have, quite arbitrarily, carried over and sought to apply within a service group under wartime

> conditions standards established under peacetime conditions within a civilian group. It is obvious on reflection, however, that the function of a psychiatrist dealing with service cases is, not to cure patients seeking relief from personal distress, but to rehabilitate sailors, soldiers and airmen who have ceased to fulfil the requirements of the group to which they belong. So far as I am personally concerned, it required little experience to discover that the problem of the war neuroses was essentially a problem of morale, i.e. a problem of the relationship of the individual member of a service to that service as a group. Thus it became obvious that the neurotic soldier was an individual who had in varying degree ceased to be a soldier in spirit—if indeed he had ever wholeheartedly accepted allegiance to the military group at all.
>
> (290)

Fairbairn is not only stating that a military doctor is obliged to the military rather than to the patient. He points to the distressed soldiers' inability to comply as itself marking a psychological, rather than a merely disciplinary, failure, hinting at a personality-wide difficulty in relating and integrating the various psychic components. Neuroses that develop around military service and war may have more to do than is initially apparent with the patients' internal makeup. These neuroses are not exclusively responses to actual combat and appear in soldiers who have never participated in the fighting. The illness, then, is not one of acute fear or sensory overload. It is, instead, an aversion to impersonal obligation that stems from preferring the attachments of private life – ultimately that of child to caregiver – over the mature dependence expected of citizens:

> An unmistakable disturbance of the personality is…involved in the development of a war neurosis. This disturbance is part and parcel of the regression involved in that revival of a hidden state of infantile dependence.
>
> (286)

For the military patient, the early household is not properly placed beneath the outer layers of civic obligation and does not nourish that obligation. On the contrary: the pull of early attachment and its representation through internal objects disrupts the patient's ability to function as an adult in an environment far removed from the caring one of the home. The neurotic soldier 'has remained…so closely identified with his original love-objects that he is incapable of establishing any stable emotional relationship with the military group' (281).

However, health resides in the ability to contain the comforting experiences of early attachment and dependence rather than in discarding them. Denying such attachments, even within the context of war, is as detrimental to mind and society alike as unduly emphasizing them. Fairbairn views overzealous militarism as pathological in the same way that evading military service through symptoms is. The two are not opposed. They are different variants on the same phenomenon. A conscript who identifies with the army to the point of denying all other associations merely transfers infantile dependence on parent and home to another object. Instead of clinging to the parent, he clings to the institution. In both cases, one observes a lack of differentiation, and an inability to contain complexity or tolerate external friction, along with a failure of mature dependence. Like the casualties of homesickness, the militarists are harmful for the purposes of the army itself. Externally conveying the impression of being 'as keen as mustard', these individuals 'are intolerant of such delays as are involved in training, become irritated by routine duties and soon begin to smart under the imagined failure of the military authorities to reward their devotion' (Fairbairn, 1952: 278). This frustration betrays an illness as acute as that of the service-evader.

Outside the extreme circumstances of war, civic commitment manifests in obeying law and adhering to the society's shared morality. Disobeying them is equivalent to evading military service. Fairbairn (1952) openly compares the 'problem of the war neuroses' to what he thinks is another form of the same phenomenon: 'similar considerations apply to those who commit unnatural sexual offences in civilian life' (290). At first, the comparison appears skewed. Etiologically, Fairbairn admits, the two are distinct. Neurotic conscripts use illness as a defence against acknowledging that a break has occurred within themselves. Having disappointed internalized social expectations, they revert to their earliest attachments and deny the later development of the personality. They pay the price of illness for a breach that they recognize committing. By contrast, sexual delinquents, as Fairbairn (1952) understands them, pay no price at all for living outside the social code. Their position involves no internal break. They enjoy their deviancy regardless of social disapproval. The overall structure of their personality does not revolt against their giving in to their drives. They are therefore psychopaths rather than neurotics (291). However, for Fairbairn, these considerations give in to another one: that of mature dependence, the recognition of one's obligation to others as separate individuals who have different interests than one's own. The sexual deviant and the neurotic soldier reach the same terminus of avoiding mature dependence by renouncing their link to society at large. The military patient evades military service, while the sexual deviant evades morality and law.

The professional response in both cases should also be similar. While, as individuals, neurotic soldiers may be treated in the clinic, collectively they present a delinquent pattern that has to be addressed as such. Fairbairn (1952) comments: 'after gaining some experience of psychoneurotic and psychotic servicemen *en masse*, I was driven to remark "what these people need is not a psychotherapist, but an evangelist'" (81). The issue, and therefore the clinical method deployed have to do with the ability to attach oneself to other people and their shared ends, rather with mending internal fractures. Group treatment, Fairbairn contends, has during the war proved more efficient in rehabilitating fatigued troops than individual therapy (295). He accordingly favours a special environment for addressing such cases, a form of institutionalization in which inmates are inculcated with collective discipline through the experience of a regulated life within a group. 'Evangelism' takes on an appropriately medical form by creating an ambience where patients can be enthused, with their emotional potential being encouraged through the experience itself. Moreover, on the symbolic level, Fairbairn thinks that soldiers who were discharged from service because of neurosis should not be awarded a war pension. While their illness is genuine and so merits compensation, its title should be differentiated from the remuneration granted to other veterans: these veterans have participated fully in the life of their society, while the neurotics have not (287–278).

Similarly, Fairbairn (1952) suggests that sexual offenders should not be approached primarily with the tools of individual psychotherapy, as they do not repress anything that the therapist may explore. The one end of treating them is implanting in them a commitment to society that will be strong enough to balance their urges. Hence, Fairbairn recommends the 'establishment of special communities for offenders...with a group life of their own, in which offenders can participate, and which is psychologically controlled with a view to its gradual approximation to the life of the community at large' (294). Dysfunctional neurotic soldiers are sent to an institution which imitates army life. Sexual offenders are sent to an institution which imitates society generally. In both cases, incarceration is training in cooperating with non-intimate and differentiated others. It is an apprenticeship in citizenship for those not currently fit for citizenship itself.

Fairbairn, then, draws a boundary between normal society, with its imperfect individuals who are marked by internal splits and are accessible to therapy, and the cluster of outcasts of various descriptions and etiologies. These are placed beyond the reach of individual therapy, and are instead regulated by institutionalized discipline calculated to ultimately allow them to turn into full participants. The underlying causes of each individual case are less important to Fairbairn than the visible outcome, and it is by the standard of this outcome that he proposes to determine policy. These exclusions are not technical details. Separating the healthy, mature and moral from its opposite and giving that separation an institutional form are constituents of Fairbairn's agenda and a consequence of the ethical motivation that propels his theory.

As for its vehicle that motivation uses Hegel along with Hegel's attitude to the state and citizenship, Fairbairn's social position differs from that offered by other object relations thinkers. Ian Suttie's notion of endogenous repression entails that a relatively tension-free venue is in principle available from infancy to adulthood. No essential split remains to constantly trouble the personality. A society made of such individuals is also reasonably tension-free, and therefore does not require a different rationale and a different set of rules than those that govern the household. Response to the child's quest for relating governs all social levels, so that most disruptions and illnesses are addressed as a deficit of relating. This included criminal behaviour. Delinquency is accordingly a proper subject of individual therapy. It does not invite formal exclusion. Delinquency, Suttie (1999) argues, is at bottom a concomitant of the culture itself rather than a pathology of the individual. It is one of the harms caused by the reduced stature of women in patriarchy, where mothers are unable to provide their children with the confidence that comes only from receiving the care of a confident parent. Feeling the deficit of relating, these children turn to violence and crime (44). As a therapeutic practice for a deeply flawed, patriarchal society, the analytic approach Suttie proposes takes the deficit of love into account, offering empathy rather than punishment to the afflicted: 'They need parental love, and its denial aggravates the need and its symptoms' (171). In a similar way, Winnicott's cartography is concentric. Home is where we start from, and whatever occurs in the home repeats elsewhere. As the dynamic of early holding is fundamentally benevolent, Winnicott assumes the possibility of a self-regulating, mainly peaceful and in principle global culture, where violence appears only as a distortion of relating, and should be managed as such. Winnicott suggests that in some cases technically criminal acts should be understood as manifesting the perpetrator's acceptance of social belonging rather than reneging on that belonging (Hopkins, 2005). Deprived of sufficient earlier care, the individual behaving in this way announces their wish to be let back into the fold by demonstrative acts: delinquency may stand for 'a moment of hope' (Winnicott, 1984: 309).

By contrast to Suttie and Winnicott, Fairbairn accepts Hegel's depiction of mind as essentially unified but inevitably split and partial. Whatever integration is available in such a world must include the mind's own recognition of its previous partiality, a move manifest by the ability to engage with a new organizational level on its own grounds and according to its own rules. Civic obligation thus differs qualitatively from the parental function which is nonetheless its necessary basis. Essential health does not show in subscription to a diffuse culture that replicates, if in varying forms, the trusting relationships of the home. It shows in obedience to impersonal regulations that contrast with the home. Crime and malingering are therefore not just deficits of function. By showing a regressive pull that demands treatment from the civic community, such acts betray a more systemic inability to accept the multilayered, dialectical character of the entire civilization. Such acts cannot be addressed as psychological or medical problems alone. Instead, they involve a moral fault, a denial of one's relative place in a world whose essence is to connect and integrate a myriad of other constituents.

Conclusion

An axial figure in the emergence of the object relations tradition, Fairbairn shares many themes with its other authors. In particular, his notion of the child as primarily object-seeking gives the sociable, other-oriented drive that Ian Suttie assumed a grounding in a structured psychoanalytical model that Fairbairn understands as resulting from an internal and logical development within psychoanalysis itself. However, Fairbairn aligns his psychology with a social vision which is not common among object relations theorists. Fairbairn understands the mind as essentially unified but also as universally divided. Acknowledging both features is a condition of health: individuals should be capable of both conceding their emotional neediness and connection to others, and function within environments which do not respect such factors, thus allowing for space where the integrated personality can fulfil itself by action. While deploying Klein's insights and some of her terms to describe the self's division into coexisting layers, Fairbairn places these insights within a Hegelian worldview which sees the family and the state as two ends of human development. The home provides the space where the pressing need for validation can be met. The civic arena, with its cold impartiality and its sometimes unforgiving demands, provides the space where the ability to externalize one's abilities and commitment can unfold. If the care and immediate attention of the parent are essential for health, then so is the horizon of adult exertion, risk and sacrifice. As in Hegel, the home setting remains crucial for Fairbairn while being placed beneath the social and political structures. Fairbairn resembles Ian Suttie and Winnicott by describing a trajectory from dependence to relative independence, but his emphasis is on independence as a goal rather than on dependence and holding as an origin. In terms of political philosophy, Fairbairn's approach entails accepting the force-wielding character of the state as a crucial feature that cannot be subsumed under or circumvented by the more peaceful, pre-political or non-political culture. In terms of policy, this leads Fairbairn, as it led Bosanquet, to distinguish citizens from outcasts and delinquents.

A well-known question in the cultural history of psychoanalysis has to do with Oedipus as a trope: what happens if we substitute Antigone for Oedipus? Replies usually converge around replacing the masculine preoccupation with castration with a more inclusive approach that focuses on relatedness (Leonard, 2013; Shainess, 1982). However, Fairbairn's revision of Freud suggests that such a move to Antigone may be more compatible with Hegel's hierarchy of family and public participation than with the vision of Antigone as a moral or political agent. *Oedipus Rex* is an investigation: why did plague come to Thebes? In Freud, this stands for the psychoanalytic process by which the individual delves into his or her emotional past for elements which disturb the present. For Hegel, by contrast, *Antigone* is not about resolving contradiction by exposing the truth. It is about relegating partial truth to a lower tier of mind and society in order to both contain it and allow us to pursue a more comprehensive truth. Kinship, for Hegel, is not denied. It is subjugated. To the extent that the argument here is correct, Fairbairn's perspective is not ultimately concerned with telling us who we are. This may be a means. The end is burying the question, letting it go, so as to make us able to engage with the world in the locations it offers us, the most developed among which is the civic arena held together by the state.

References

Beaney, T. (2009). Beautiful death: The nineteenth century fascination with Antigone. *Opticon* 1826 (7): 1–8.

Benjamin, J. (1999). Recognition and destruction: An outline of intersubjectivity. In Mitchell, S.A., and Aron, L. (eds.), *Relational psychoanalysis: The emergence of a tradition*. Hillsdale, NJ: The Analytic Press, 181–210.

Birtles, E.F. (2002). Why is Fairbairn relevant today – A modernist/postmodernist view. In Pereira, F., and Scharff, D.E. (eds.), *Fairbairn and relational theory*. London: Karnac, 36–52.

Birtles, E. Fairbairn (2005). Difference, repetition and continuity: Philosophical reflections on Fairbairn's concept of mature dependence. In Scharff, J.S., and Scharff, D.E. (eds.), *The legacy of Fairbairn and Sutherland*. London and New York: Routledge, 39–49.

Bosanquet, B. (1910). Charity organization and the Majority Report. *International Journal of Ethics* 20 (4): 395–408.

Bosanquet, B. (2001). *The philosophical theory of the state*. Kitchener: Batoche.

Bradley, J. (1979). Hegel in Britain: A brief history of British commentary and attitudes. *The Heynthrop Journal* 20 (1): 1–24.

Brooks, T. (2007). *Hegel's political philosophy*. Edinburgh: Edinburgh University Press.

Clarke, G.S. (2006). *Personal relations theory*. Hove: Routledge.

Clarke, G.S. (2011). Suttie's influence on Fairbairn's object relations theory. *Journal of the American Psychoanalytic Association* 59 (5): 939–959.

Den Otter, S. (1996). *British idealism and social explanation*. Oxford: Oxford University Press.

Fairbairn, N. (1987). *A life is too short*, London: Quartet.

Fairbairn, R.W.D. (1994). *From instinct to self*. London: Jason Aronson.

Fairbairn, W.R.D. (1952). *Psycho-analytic studies of the personality*. London: Tavistock.

Franco, P. (1997). Hegel and liberalism. *The Review of Politics* 59 (4): 831–860.

Grotstein, J.S. (2000). Notes on Fairbairn's metapsychology. In Grotstein, J.S., and Rinsley, D.B. (eds.), *Fairbairn and the origins of object relations*. New York: Other Press, 112–148.

Guntrip, H. (1961). *Personality structure and human interaction.* New York: International Universities Press.

Hegel, G.W.F. (1952). *Hegel's philosophy of right.* Oxford: Clarendon.

Honig, B. (2013). *Antigone interrupted.* Cambridge: Cambridge University Press.

Hopkins, B. (2005). Winnicott and imprisonment. *American Imago* 62 (3): 269–283.

Kernberg, O.F. (2000). Fairbairn's theory and challenge. In Grotstein, J.S., and Rinsley, D.B. (eds.), *Fairbairn and the origins of object relations.* New York: Other Press, 41–65.

Kernberg, O.F. (2002). A contemporary exploration of the contributions of W.R.D. Fairbairn. In Pereira, F., and Scharff, D.E. (eds.), *Fairbairn and relational theory.* London: Karnac, 11–27.

Leonard, M. (2013). Freud and tragedy: Oedipus and the gender of the universal. *Classical Receptions Journal* 5 (1): 63–83.

Levy, J. (2014). Fairbairn's unique contributions to dream interpretation. In Clarke, G.S., and Scharff, D.E. (eds.), *Fairbairn and the object relations tradition.* London: Karnac, 237–248.

Miller, G. (2008). Scottish psychoanalysis: A rational religion. *Journal of the History of the Behavioral Sciences* 44 (1): 38–59.

Mitchell, S.A. (2000). The origin and nature of the 'object' in the theories of Klein and Fairbairn. In Grotstein, J.S., and Rinsley, D.B. (eds.), *Fairbairn and the origins of object relations.* New York: Other Press, 66–87.

Morrow, J. (1984), Liberalism and British idealist political philosophy: A reassessment. *History of Political Thought* 5 (1): 91–108.

Nicholson, P.P. (1990). *The political philosophy of the British idealists.* Cambridge: Cambridge University Press.

Ogden, T.H. (1992). *The matrix of the mind: Object relations and the psychoanalytic dialogue.* London: Karnac.

Ogden, T.H. (2010). Why read Fairbairn? *International Journal of Psychoanalysis* 91: 101–118.

Scharff, D.E. (2005). The development of Fairbairn's theory. In Scharff, J.S., and Scharff, D.E. (eds.), *The legacy of Fairbairn and Sutherland.* London and New York: Routledge, 3–18.

Shainess, N. (1982). Antigone, the neglected daughter of Oedipus: Freud's gender concepts in theory. *Journal of the American Academy of Psychoanalysis*, 10 (3): 443–455.

Sharpe, C. (2016). From the individual, to the relational and communal: The Kirk's influence on three Scottish thinkers: Ronald Fairbairn, John Macmurray and Ian Suttie. *Ethics and Social Welfare* 10 (3): 224–238.

Suttie, I.D. (1999). *The origins of love and hate.* New York: Julian.

Winnicott, D.W. (1984). *Through paediatrics to psychoanalysis.* London: Karnac.

Winnicott, D.W. (1986). *Home is where we start from.* New York: Norton.

Winnicott, D.W. (1991). *Playing and reality.* London: Routledge.

4 Donald Winnicott

Transition to Liberty

Winnicott's work has a nearly unmatched span and breadth. His theory is as innovative and tightly structured as Fairbairn's, while his commitment to a comprehensive philosophy that asks what our entire lives are about is as strong as Ian Suttie's. Winnicott grounds a social optimism comparable to that of Suttie within a methodological basis and a terminology that draws from Klein. The dour tone of Klein's model itself is allayed by Winnicott's endorsement of an object-seeking drive, as in Fairbairn. The outcome is a worldview which is at once individualistic and liberal, but is nonetheless anchored to a reassuring social framework that prioritizes closeness and emotional validation. These issues have been touched on in biographical works by Jacobs (1988), Kahr (1996), Phillips (1988) and Rodman (2003). Alexander (2012) and Nussbaum (2006) place Winnicott within the intellectual context of an expanding and enriched concern with personal freedom. I have previously discussed Winnicott in similar terms, pointing to his compatibility with the notions of welfare entitlement and deliberation (Gerson, 2005, 2017). Here, I point to the places where Winnicott's ideas match the combination of liberal ideas effected by the welfare-state thought of the early to middle twentieth century, in the sense of anticipating an influx of habits and norms from the healthy privacy of the home into the public sphere.

Health and Integration

Subscribing to the Kleinian terminology, Winnicott understands maternal presence as the organizing factor of infantile personality. He is likewise interested in the dialectic of aggression and reparation that is central to Klein's work. However, Winnicott's different set of attitudes and experiences register in his offering a theory that does not simply replicate Klein. Unlike Klein, Winnicott emphasizes the real mother and focuses on the child's actual interaction with her, substituting Klein's preoccupation with imaginary objects. While Klein recognizes internal objects and external objects, Winnicott's trademark innovation is the third realm, the transitional space populated by transitional phenomena and transitional objects (Greenberg and Mitchell, 1983: 201–205; Phillips, 1988: 45–47).

Unlike the imaginary persecuting breast or the real caring mother, the transitional object is both internal and external. The transitional object – the blanket or soft toy the child clings to – is a tangible item that may be observed by others. At the same time, it is invested by the child with subjective meaning. For the child, the blanket or toy has a reassuring presence and an identity of its own: it cannot be swapped with just any other identically looking item. This makes the object a significant presence in family life, an external addition to the child's personality. The child thus creates an object that has already been there for all to see. Relationship with the object differs by virtue of its tangibility from solipsistic fantasying, while at the same time it differs from passive compliance with reality by effecting a change, making a mass of matter meaningful and personal. Later, play, sports, literature, art, music and other cultural forms occupy the space originally filled with the blanket or toy: they are all shared illusions, subjective creations that are yet out there for others to perceive. When performance of adult tasks involves more than mechanic repetition, it requires a sense of personal meaning invested in the act. Such performance therefore occurs in the transitional space that originates with the infantile use of blanket or toy (Winnicott, 1991: 95–103).

To create such an object, the child needs to have an idea of comfort and warmth to project onto it, and a basic confidence that frees him or her to explore and create. Both conditions depend on earlier parental care. Enjoying an initial illusion of omnipotence through having their wishes attended to, infants will have already gained confidence in their creative powers by the time they realize the existence of a limiting external reality. When, inevitably, the parent 'fails' the child by tuning down the immediate and close attention that had been necessary in earliest infancy, the child is led to recognize the independent existence of the parent. The child endures this recognition because of the reassuring image internalized in the earlier phase, of which the unique status given to the blanket or toy is a projection. The space opened up between parent and infant is where the transitional object lives. It is a gap inhabited by processed memories of wholeness (Winnicott, 1991: 1–25). Reliable parenting thus involves both close care and the capacity to instil acknowledgement of separation. Once the potential space opens up, the caregiver demonstrates their recognition of the child's needs by respecting the transitional object and avoiding challenging the child's perception of the object as special and meaningful.

The notion of transition has implications beyond childcare. Winnicott is clear that whatever happens in the smallest social unit – the nursing dyad, mother and child – structures the broader levels of social organization. The capacity to use transitional space depends on the relationship with the parent but, in turn, allows for further relationships. The original, gradual distancing from minute care allows the child to create the object that, as it is out there to be seen by others, constitutes a means of communication. Consequently, distance from others is experienced as a bridge to them. The realization of separateness harbours the possibility of dialogue. 'In ever-widening circles of social life', Winnicott (1965b: 91) writes, 'the child is identified with society, because local society is a sample of the self's personal world as well as being a truly external phenomenon'.

Independent personhood, then, is, for Winnicott, an end rather than a premise. Winnicott (1965b: 57) finds 'no value whatever in describing babies in the earliest stages except in relation to the mother's functioning'. This statement relates to more than physical dependence. It means that people's identities, their each having a sense of difference from others, depend on others' attention. Individual mind cannot be understood and analyzed outside a social context. The simple act of recognizing our own distinct identity by gazing into a mirror echoes the infant's look into the mother's face, a quest for *social* assurance (Winnicott, 1991: 111–118). Initially, the baby is an aggregate of sensations and body parts that require an external presence if they are to integrate. The anchor provided by the parent's consistent attention allows the various inputs that go into the making of individuality – fantasy and somatic stimuli, past, present and future – to crystallize into a tolerably cohesive whole: 'all these parts are gathered together by the mother who is holding the child' (Winnicott, 1989: 568). The presence of an integrated self tells of prior socialization. Conversely, the absence of the other amounts to absence of self.

Enabling the distinct and integrated personality to eventually surface, however, remains Winnicott's desired end. Winnicott (1965b: 29–36) argues that 'the capacity to be alone' is a consequence of being with someone. The child first plays in the presence of the mother, whose 'holding' allows play: the other's presence guarantees the self's own survival, thus providing conditions for relaxation. Later, the actual mother may be substituted by a symbol, such as a cot, leaving the child alone. The environment's assurance has been internalized to a degree that actual care is no longer urgent. One manifests one's trust in others, therefore, by being capable of separating from them. Being alone is presented by Winnicott as a *capacity*: it is a token of confidence, proving that the child feels real and whole enough to stop the constant look to others for signs of approval. Healthy individuals are both linked to others and differentiate from them, as these are two aspects of the same healthy existence (Winnicott, 1965b: 83). Accordingly, Winnicott (1986: 65–70) leaves space for both the socially visible, surface persona he calls the false self, and the subjective depth he calls the true self. The two have to communicate if the personality is to remain ultimately integrated: both dissociation between the hidden and visible parts of the personality and the suppression or denial of any of them are pathological (Winnicott, 1991: 68–70, 79–84, 86–94).

Alongside its socially conditioned nature, Winnicott anchors individuality in structured social settings and in the division of tasks and the hierarchies that they involve. To realize one's separate existence and the communicative possibilities of transitional space, one first needs to experience, and make good use of, the reassuring presence of another person. In infancy, the parent provides this basic presence, and in treatment, the therapist. The relationship within each such pair is fundamentally unequal. The parent or therapist provides the reliability that the child or patient does not find within. The integration of personality that arises from successful parenting or clinical work is accordingly conditional upon the existence of a power differential between parent and child, therapist and patient. Health depends on the more vulnerable partner's 'capacity to believe in getting help and to trust the one who offers help' (Winnicott, 1989: 299). Therapists should therefore operate within 'a strictly professional setting in which the patient is free to explore' (Winnicott, 1989: 299). The analyst regulates contact and makes his or her availability temporally and spatially fixed. These attributes serve to broadcast authority and reliability. While Winnicott assures his patients of their value for others, such assurances derive their force from being made by an expert at his office. Authority heals people and makes them feel real and whole. The inequality of parent and child, holder and held, therapist and patient, enables individuals to retain their separate personhood and connect to other individuals, even while it does all this by disseminating egalitarian messages (Winnicott, 1986: 96–97, 1989: 279). Multifaceted but integrated, healthy agents act in the space that connects their own subjectivity with those of others while accepting differentiation in social roles and positions as part of the enabling environment.

Disrupted integration defines most illness. When the capacity to play does not fully mature, the paranoid-schizoid layer of the personality remains dominant. The other is not a person to be related to, but a collection of persecuting objects to be defended against. As infantile dependence does not permit the child to rebel in reality, the relationship with the parent, and later with reality, consists in compliance. Ill agents dissociate their social from their introspective selves, manifesting the schizoid nature of most pathology. The crust-like false self is tasked with functioning within a reality that is too unsafe for the submerged kernel self to face (Winnicott, 1965b: 58–60, 145–147). Mechanically conforming to external demands and apparently giving up their private illusions, personalities impacted in this way indulge their illusions in some hidden recess of the mind, thus assuring that illusions are what they remain. As social engagement is detached from internal being, it is experienced as caving in, fostering resentment and barring the individual from trusting the stronger, parental and therapeutic agents, on whose care a healthier sense of agency depends. Like fantasy, whatever resentment and aggression accumulate in such minds cannot find an outlet in the real world. Individuals structured like this develop a matching perception of themselves and the world, in which authenticity and personal meaning are understood as opposed to engagement with others. However, as personal distinction and the sensation of creativity rely on the other's internalized or actual validation, such an internally partitioned personality is gradually depleted, to the point of its owner having little perception of themselves as an individual. As one patient reports, 'I have been playing patience … in my empty room and the room is really empty because while I am playing patience I do not exist' (Winnicott, 1991: 36).

Personal Entitlement in the Social Order

The high normative value Winnicott places on achieving a sense of integrated, complex and socially engaged individuality; the dependence of this achievement on society and its structures; and the institutional settlement entailed by his work all concur with liberal theory and with the twentieth century's synthesis of historical liberal variants. Winnicott's view of internally differentiated, biologically grounded social bonds as the necessary bedrock of individuality echoes Locke's view of natural society as the normative benchmark to which the state should be accountable. Winnicott provides ammunition to the liberal emphasis on the benevolence of, and consequently the entitlement owed to, the private sphere by showing that tensions within it are not necessarily destructive. Like the initial 'failure' of the parent to respond that triggers the opening up of transitional space, frustration of social expectations may contribute to the process through which we both acknowledge each other and maintain our mutual distinction. The private realm based on the initial bond and the supportive family contains friction as a necessary, ultimately constructive part of itself. Accordingly, while Winnicott to an extent shares Marx's or Foucault's perception of individuality as constructed by economic and power structures, he differs normatively from these authors because he views such construction as potentially benevolent (Alford, 2000: 251; Flax, 1990: 110, 116, 1993a: 17; Hoggett, 1992: 11–20). He accordingly neither condemns the marks of socialization that the person carries as oppressive branding, nor argues for dismantling individuality itself. While valuing spontaneity, Winnicott (1986: 65–70) perceives a measured presence of the false self as essential for healthy functioning and as pointing to the individual's ability to recognize objective reality. A degree of alienation and role-playing alongside the required functional inequality is thus inevitable, and Winnicott does not envisage overcoming such forms of inauthenticity by transforming production structures. Winnicott's idea of individuality as both enabled and valued by society affiliates with Locke's and Mill's liberalism rather than with the radicalism of Marx or Foucault.

By favouring individuality as a normative end while acknowledging its necessary basis in social structuring, Winnicott approaches an individualist perception of rights as immunities against social intervention.

In the liberal tradition, the entitlement to hold on to a possession is a paradigmatic right because property makes the immunity included in the concept of rights concrete, embodying it in physical objects. Liberals such as Locke (1946: 15–16) emphasize the exclusive character of property. Eating is necessary for human survival, so that respecting everyone's ability to do it obligates us if we concede that everyone is entitled to live. As anything once eaten cannot be used by others, accepting it as a right entails that we respect property in the sense of something held away by the individual. If J.S. Mill (1977: 229–257, 272–274) contests Locke's attribution of rights' origins to the natural state, he predicates them on utility: the liberty of doing whatever does not harm others is instrumental for enlarging the pool of ideas that society may use. Again, a certain range of actions is placed beyond society's discretion and becomes the exclusive mandate of each right-holding individual.

Winnicott combines these perceptions. Rights indeed involve unquestioned immunity, but they mutually benefit the society that grants them. On the one hand, our most pressing need is sharing and communicating rather than excluding. Beyond its instrumental value for personal integration, sharing meanings with others is, for Winnicott, one of the goods enjoyed by the integrated personality. Whatever renders life worth living – literature, music, sports – takes place in transitional space (Winnicott, 1991: 99, 105). Such activities consist in the externalization of abilities, inclinations and ideas. Their value is derived from their ability to make the subjective and internal available to others. The communicative potential they include is emotionally rewarding, and therefore therapeutic, like nothing else. That reward does not necessitate actual company. The drive for painting, composing music or performing drama may require only the internalized image of the parent, possibly compiled into a social or religious symbol. Hiding or denying the inclination to reach out through such channels amounts to auto-excommunication, which is a major source of pain as well as a potential source of social disruption. Humans are consumed by guilt and self-fulfilling fears when having no space in which to meet their fellows (Winnicott, 1991: 68–90). Transitional space serves as the location of communication, the place where subjective interpretations converse: the child's view of the teddy with the parent's, my idea of fine art with yours. Rights, accordingly, are valued for enabling participation.

But they function by making individuals immune to others' intervention in particular places, thus placing an obligation on these others to stand away. Property, again, serves as the paradigmatic right, as evidenced by the terminology Winnicott (1991) uses for describing what takes place in transitional space. The transitional object is the 'first possession' (1–2). While inseparable from the child's persona, the blanket or toy is still an objective phenomenon that is not a part of the child's body. While none but the child may use it, everyone perceives it. Transitional objects are created when parental support has been internalized to such a degree that it can be projected onto an object and maintained even when the actual parent is absent. Hence, the ability to appropriate signifies the appropriator's mooring in prior care. The right and the property one is entitled to use according to one's discretion are a shared illusion that should not be challenged, like the child's special blanket, the book, the game or the concert (Flax, 1993b: 343).

This perception of right and property may also be approached through its obverse in destruction and theft. For Winnicott, failure in the development of transitional capacities indicates a failure of care. When the internal representation of the parent is partially lost, the child is unable to project it onto the environment (Winnicott, 1991: 20–25). The search for the lost object is then manifested in stealing real objects. Having lost faith in parental care and, consequently, having lost the internal representation of the parent, the delinquent is driven by a compulsion to retrieve it. Stealing is aimed not at the good's financial value, but at the link it offers to the outside (Winnicott, 1984: 125). For Winnicott, having assured access to anything, legitimate or stolen, is participation: a relation to society, not a defence against it or a space enclosed from it.

Winnicott (1991) further reflects liberal philosophy by shoring up the necessity of constitution and the rule of law. When the child distinguishes self from environment, subjectivity and objectivity are differentiated, and, in between them, transitional space opens up for the dynamics of play and the many activities based on it. But if transitional space is open, both the individual's body and external reality are not (106–107). For transitional space to form, the individual has first to acknowledge corporeal and external reality. There is no meaningful movement without a confining boundary: the soft toy has to be out there first for the infant to create it as a meaningful transitional object; games need a ball, a court, a set of rules; literature requires language; art requires an audience that has some concept of art into which to fit the artist's unique contribution. Recognition of such structures is play's condition. If some meanings are open to negotiation, other meanings have to be fixed and reside beyond negotiation. Recognizing the existence of an external reality either in its physical sense of a given cosmos or in the social sense of obligating rule is also the source of the capacity to feel concern for others. Driven by apparently aggressive though pre-moral stimuli, the infant pushes, nudges and bites the mother's body. As the mother survives these attacks, the infant realizes the existence of facts outside his or her control. At the same time, the mother's survival minimizes the significance of the attacks and so makes the infant capable of tolerating his or her own aggression, owning up to it and desiring to compensate for it. Thus, acknowledgement of one's limited control over reality and concern for others are acquired at the same moment (86–94). Similarly, in the clinical setting, providing patients with a stable sense of reality is curative. Tuning down the constricting potential of logical objectivity by minimizing clinical interpretation, Winnicott would rather help patients make their own interpretations by providing them with the strict setting established by the time limit and the professional legitimation. Within this structured environment, the patient develops a secure subjectivity, which may then be mined and discussed with the therapist. Clinical dialogue depends on the order maintained by the analyst. But to do this, the clinician has to be processed by the patient as a real other person who is beyond the patient's control, or the dialogue will remain internal and fantastic (87). The temporal limitations of the consultation, its location and its overall structure are all aspects of the analyst's function as an objective phenomenon. Consequently, Flax writes that, for Winnicott, 'without pregiven structures...no creativity would be possible' (1993b: 339).

Institutions and Public Guidelines

Winnicott, then, reflects historical liberalism's advocacy of recognizing individuals' need for having a space apart for themselves, and that liberalism's trust in a structured order with known patterns and rules. Winnicott reflects his time's liberal turn towards the welfare state by advocating certain legal and policy guidelines for safeguarding the tenets of individual immunity to intervention of the rule of law. Winnicott describes individuality as arising from parental adjustment. First, the illusion of omnipotence secures coherence and confidence, and, when this has been achieved, gradual separation alerts the child to the rift between self and other. Therapy repeats this pattern. Often, it begins with maximal adjustment to the patient's needs so as to allow a period of relaxation, dependence and confidence-building. Then, gradually, the therapist begins to 'fail' and so organizes the patient into recognition of distance. This subsequently enables real communication based on the acknowledgement of the therapist's separate existence. Such a relationship does not necessarily require professional knowledge. It may be initiated by psychological laity such as teachers and bureaucrats: results are achieved by the structure of the relationship more than by its content. In each social location, individualities are moulded by the subsequent stages of close attention and gradual distancing. On all levels, the confidence generated by the holding environment enables individuals to negotiate their distance from others through the manifold channels offered by transitional phenomena (Winnicott, 1986: 96–97).

The organization of government and its agencies follows on this view. Winnicott (1986: 240–241) argues that democracy is conditioned on the nuclear family. To be capable of playing and participating, a certain psychological package is needed, which can form only within a secure environment: 'full maturity for the individual is not possible in an immature or ill social setting' (1965b: 84). This is related to the question of tolerance in a complex society. Individuality and separateness produce a variety of viewpoints. These can only take root and become meaningful when other people tolerate them. These other individuals, in their turn – parents, therapists, siblings and peers – are rendered tolerant by confidence in their own integration, which is itself dependent on ample parenting. A certain type of family is essential for establishing such confidence: heterosexual and functionally divided. Crucial for the growth of the integrated personality is close care by a specific person who can maintain steady proximity to the infant and adjust to its needs. Without close attention, the infant would not be able to develop the comforting and stabilizing internal images needed for personal integration. Such conditions are best provided by the infant's natural parents in their own home: a mother to care for the child, and a father to act as 'the protecting agent who frees the mother to devote herself to her baby' (1986: 248). The parents as a team, moreover, have to feel safe from arbitrary pressures, so as not to be distracted from their respective tasks. If democracy needs nuclear families, such families in their turn cannot thrive under tyranny. They require the immune space created by legal rights to insulate them from the outside. Addressing the problem of strengthening democracy in the aftermath of the Second World War, Winnicott suggests that democracy should be based on unimpeded nuclear families. Government must essentially 'avoid interfering with the homes that can cope' (Winnicott, 1986: 246).

Furthermore, the family as a unit merits active help in order to maintain its basic structure. Society should safeguard the home's viability by putting resources at its disposal (Winnicott, 1965a: 114–120). These resources, in the shape of social services and national insurance, function to render the male breadwinner more confident about his place in the world. This confidence, in its turn, makes easier the wife's task of concentrating on the child. If the family is the child's facilitating environment, then society, through its welfare apparatus, should be the family's facilitating environment: 'social provision is very much an extension of the family' (93). At all organizational levels, Winnicott suggests protecting individuals from the intense pressures of reality in order to make them eventually capable of enduring, and acting independently within, this reality. Power is charged with defending individuals from acute insecurity. Freed from the anxiety involved in such insecurity, the individual finds the confidence to be truly creative instead of merely compliant. Welfare measures screen the more volatile aspects of the market away from private lives, and so generate the risk-taking, explorative economic player: capitalism depends on socialism, the free market on regulation.

If the organization of the good society follows and complements the principles of good parenting, then this means that the space opened up for the family by government should be likewise secured and delimited by government. Democracy, Winnicott (1986: 240) thinks, should be defined by its attention to the needs of its healthier members: the polity safeguards their potentiality for agency and creativity. Democracy, then, should primarily respect the privacy of individuals and the family home where the capacity for agency can form (Winnicott, 1991: 109). In one of its aspects, then, democracy is committed to keeping power away from the sites of privacy. But democracy also has a more proactive function. As health is largely determined by environmental responses to the child, it is an environmental responsibility. Just as the family is the environment of the child, society is the environment of the family, entailing 'a need to make society acknowledge and repay' when families are distressed (Winnicott, 1965b: 207). Such acknowledgement manifests as preventative, educative and restorative services. Homes, Winnicott (1986: 247) writes, 'need all that science can offer in respect of physical health and the prevention and treatment of physical disease; they also want instruction in child care, and help when their children have psychological illnesses or present behaviour problems'. Taken together, the state's commitment to keeping away from privacy and its corresponding obligation to aid and foster private sites add up to a welfare state based on liberal premises.

The obverse of the concern with the autonomy of the household is potential monitoring of its structure. Taking place within families, the parenting activity that is essential for a good society might occasionally be insufficient in practice, possibly because of circumstances among which Winnicott (1986: 247) numbers parents who are unmarried or divorced. Such parents cannot afford the time and attention involved in the intense adjustment infants require, and do not always enable the maturation of the confident personality. Accordingly, Winnicott (1965a: 109–110) urges medical, nursing and social-work staff to address the difficulties of the mother who is 'immature, or not orientated to the part the woman plays in nature's comic opera; or who is perhaps depressed, anxious, suspicious, or just muddled'. Exposing the household's interior to the official gaze is a device meant to cultivate the democratic personality that can withstand other individuals. While it cushions individuals against economic pressures and so aids them in running secure homes, the state exerts its power to mould the home into compatibility with a specific social vision.

Winnicott, then, perceives individuality as produced by society rather than as simply given, but posits that securing the conditions for individuality to emerge is the cherished goal. He views engagement with others in society and culture as an extension of play with transitional objects, and would describe rights as transitional phenomena whose primacy for the individual should not be challenged even while they are known to depend on the environment's cooperation. Winnicott would have society preserve the autonomy of the home, yet surround it with a network of institutions offering professional aid and harbouring the possibility of monitoring and intervention in the life of the home. Throughout, Winnicott values the stabilizing presence of structured institutions as conducive to the emergence of the coherent personality. These ideas concur with the welfare-state project advocated by early and mid-twentieth century liberals as a response to the particular pressures of the time.

Household Tasks and Psychic Components

Setting now on a more critical survey of Winnicott's social and political implications, I address two issues: the persistence of gender roles in Winnicott's theory, and the diminishing significance he attributes to the political and civic sphere. The two points are interconnected: as constituents of a benign natural society, gender identities are not implicated by power relationships; and as that natural society can, when allowed scope, inform the political realm, that realm forfeits some of its uniqueness.

I will discuss gender first. Winnicott may to some extent be counted as aligned with a feminist critique of the gender hierarchy. By following Klein, he accepts the mother's role as the primary factor in the psyche's formation. Klein's work substitutes Freud's paternal imagery – the phallus and the castration anxiety – by a maternal imagery that involves nurture and holding. Instead of seeing femininity as consisting in lack and resentment, Klein opens up the possibility of viewing femininity as active and influential (Greenberg and Mitchell, 1983: 122–127). The mother emerges as the first and most significant person the child knows. By the oedipal stage, the child has already internalized notions taken from his relationship with the mother. Recognition of maternal agency precedes any perception of male power. But Winnicott transcends Klein here. By considering families in the flesh, a point of view enabled by his professional experience, Winnicott transforms the mother from a phantasmic object to a real person (Rustin, 1991: 26–27). This allows Winnicott to recognize women's role in shaping society. Their interests, desires, anxieties and mental makeup can no longer be ignored, as they have been for long by psychological and other social theory (Minsky, 1996; Rudnytsky, 2002).

However, Winnicott's record is not unambiguous. As a social theory that assumes that health is the default option and thus establishes an equivalent of Locke's state of nature, Winnicott's scheme places a benchmark by which all politics should be judged. That benchmark is based on apparently natural, biological processes and groupings. The inequalities of these groupings are placed beyond political enquiry and are made the basis of legitimate politics itself. While Freud traced pathology back to pressures that are integral to this family organization – the child's realization that his parents share an intimacy in which he has no part – Winnicott, along with Ian Suttie and Jane Suttie, locates the origins of ill health in intrusions on this family, such as those caused by wartime separation or the demands of the workplace. If the family normally and naturally consists of two genders and two generations, then retaining this structure equates with individual and social health. Clinicians are tasked with advising mothers who, isolated by the privacy needed to fulfil their special function, are not accessible to other interactions. Medical examination and counsel thus reinforce the family structure that Winnicott identifies with health (Jacobs, 1988: 108–114). In the course of its work, psychotherapy acts to define women's correct social position for them. Mothers become 'objects for the regulatory discourse of experts' who expect the home to organize along correct gender lines (Doane and Hodges, 1992: 21). Winnicott thereby joins an overall trend, prominent in the culture of the midcentury, of experts pronouncing on the correct conduct and life-choices of women and subtly burdening mothers with the weight of the entire society's well-being (Eyer, 1992: 110–128; Riley, 1983; Shapira, 2013: 13–18, 112–137).

Doane and Hodges (1992: 14) link Winnicott's essentialist view of gender to his methodological departure from Klein. In Klein, the infant does not relate to real people but to phantasmic objects. These may have gendered characters, but they need not be neatly sorted out. The infant may perceive the mother as having a penis, for example. When Winnicott modifies Klein, the essential difference between the sexes remains, but is moved outside, to the tangible world. The issue is no longer that of relating to shifting figures that may display any set of characters. One is on firm ground with clearly differentiated identities. By accepting their implications, individuals, and particularly women, contribute to the healthy social order. In the course of sufficient caring, the infant first enjoys the mother's unconditional attention, thus gaining the confidence to create as well as an inner notion of comfort and trust. Acquiring the empowering ability to play depends on initial undisturbed and finely tuned attention to the child's needs. This requires a parent exclusively specializing in parenting. Nurture, Winnicott writes, 'is immensely simplified if the infant is cared for by one person' (1975: 153). That single person should herself be isolated from other concerns, so as not to be distracted. 'Enjoy letting other people look after the world while you are producing a new one of its members', Winnicott (1950: 8) advises mothers. While becoming isolated, the caring parent is made economically dependent on non-carers. While Winnicott (1986: 248) prescribes seclusion for the caring parent, he advises the other parent to act as 'the protecting agent who frees the mother to devote herself to her baby'. Colluding with the gender distinction is therefore tantamount to a lucid perception of reality, as contrasted with the paranoid-schizoid world of chaotic part objects, and is at the same time functional for everybody's well-being.

It might be countered at this stage that Winnicott's perception of gender is more nuanced than the above implies. Winnicott (1986: 37, 1991: 79–80) rejects appeals, such as those made by Bowlby, to physical biology and evolution. Instead, he is entrenched within psychoanalysis, with its focus on verbalization, narrative and subjectivity. Accordingly, Winnicott (1971: 362) plays down the technical – and specifically gendered – details of childcare, such as breast feeding, and criticizes other authors, like Bowlby and Spock, for doing the opposite. Gender is therefore not a deterministic, biological essence. Instead, Winnicott views gender as different modes of differentiating self from other. Each person experiences both modes, making gender a more fluid term than may be initially assumed. All children are capable of both identifying with the mother's holding posture, and perceiving her as an object external to the self. Winnicott (1991: 79–84) refers to these two possibilities as 'being the breast' and 'using the breast'. While girls emphasize the first mode and boys the second, traces of both options remain with all individuals. As health is associated with integration, this also applies to the ability to contain and acknowledge opposite-gender identities within the self. Shorn of their link to biological attributes, the names feminine and masculine may become no more than tags attached to a mental reality that is independent of traditional identities.

As males have the same experience of early care as females, they too may become carers, which applies even to their public, supposedly impersonal, personas. As the experience of early nurture is universal, the principle of nurture repeats throughout society. At all levels of organization, individuals require reliable holding if they are to thrive independently. For example, Winnicott (1986: 90–100) counsels the principals of penitentiary schools – presumably, men used to confrontation – to treat their more troublesome charges in a way that replicates the technique of mothering. They should, Winnicott advises, set up regular individual meetings with these inmates. The contents of the sessions are less important than the principal's rigorous keeping to schedule, always being present in his office at the appointed hour. This technique is designed to generate trust and confidence in individuals who are shown by the fact of being delinquents to lack such trust and confidence. The mother and the breast are names for methods that need not have any gendered attribute.

If Winnicott is viewed mainly with this non-essential perception of gender in mind, then some of the earlier-mentioned equations of women with a specialized, homebound and economically dependent maternal function may be laid aside as period pieces. Gender can be then seen as a more dynamic and interchanging set of configurations within the object world. However, the duality of being and using, holding and being held, cannot be transcended because of the infant's indelible original dependence on, and illusion of control over, the mother. Without these conditions, babies do not acquire the confidence and relatedness of transitional space. A phase of life is always there in the mind, in which the two roles are distinct. Consequently, these two roles are constituents of the fundamental, molecular inventory out of which personalities are constituted.

They equate with the two genders and are intuitively recognizable by all as such. When a patient draws a squiggle composing a round form and a conical one that seems to burst out of the other form rather than to penetrate it, Winnicott (1971: 189) reports,

> I just simply said 'Let's leave it at that. It looks to me like the male and female principles'. She understood what I meant here and was pleased to leave it.

As the two gender elements are distinct and irreducible, individuals may not fuse or transcend them. One may be predominantly either male or female. This feeds into the notion of transitional space as the solid, objective and limiting confine within which play takes place. Satisfactory sexuality depends on the recognition of the distance between the sexes. Partners should acknowledge each other's fundamental sexual alterity. Only when this distance is recognized may it be filled with the play of shared pursuits and commitments. Resisting these insights – denying the essential division into two genders – indicates immaturity and forecloses the potentiality for play, thereby undermining the fulfilling content of conjugal relationships. Winnicott (1989: 41) interprets a patient's concern with his romantic partner's professional achievements as reflecting a hindrance to their relations, as it subtly constructs her as a male and betrays the patient's 'inability to think of a girl as different from a man because it raised his own fears of loss of penis'.

Moreover, sexuality would not be the source of reward it is unless it involved giving up on choice at certain points. As in the overall pattern of play's dependence on respect for solid boundaries, romantic relationships benefit from their ability to both be creative and concede a facet of objective reality. The reward gained from the meeting of two differing sexual identities is linked to their hinting at the Malthusian realities of reproduction and the constraint of earning a lifeline. Commenting on the mass dissemination of contraceptives in the 1960s, Winnicott accuses the pill of turning sex from an unchangeable reality connected with hard choices and therefore with commitment and responsibility, into a magical satisfaction of wishes that replicates the infantile illusion of omnipotence. Once the illusion is entered upon, real engagement with others is given up. Sexuality has to retain its implication of constraint – a constituent of a timeless natural order that involves the cycle of life and the biological vulnerabilities incurred through it – if it is to ground the satisfactory mutuality that touches and transforms the participants (Winnicott, 1986: 195–209).

The familiar two-generations, two-genders home is the institutional implementation of these insights, as it maintains the matrix of roles and functions on the basis of which relationships between the parents, and between parents and children, can unfold. Ideologically wishing to challenge this vision is itself a disruption. Winnicott's perception of feminism as a social movement is coloured by this identification of health with acceptance of gendered differentiation. Feminism, Winnicott (1986: 189–190) claims, attempts to annul the distance between wish and reality. For that reality feminism tries to substitute a world in which all individuals are endowed with the same capabilities and the same personality structure, and have therefore little need for projecting their fantasies onto each other: a wholly public, civic world without an underlying plain of interaction that reflects the original order of things and allows genuine play. For Winnicott, then, the gender distinction gains a naturalistic, imperative character. It cannot be legitimately changed by appeal to notions of equality, power sharing, domination and liberation from it.

The Expanding Realm of Play

Winnicott's attitude to gender reveals the strength of the naturalistic layer in his worldview. Its existence and character impact Winnicott's perception of politics. Along with the contents of the parental function, the gender distinction is placed in a pristine space prior to scrutiny and contest. That space is not just static. It cultivates creativity and movement. As the normative social good is grounded in that space and that space is expanding, it has the potentiality to at least partially displace politics.

This horizon is implied in the premises of Winnicott's particular take on psychoanalytic theory. He combines Ian Suttie's normative perspective with Klein's two-positions model, generating, in the shape of transitional space and transitional activities, a mechanism by which the paranoid-schizoid position is safely left behind, if never wholly dispensed with. The uniqueness of this view may stand out better when Winnicott is compared with Fairbairn.

Overall, Fairbairn's thought manifests the impact of Hegel's philosophy (Scharff, 2005). In Hegel (1952), conceding one's relativity is gratifying because it creates the possibility of recognition by another human. Set on asserting its wholeness, the self encounters resistance from others, who see themselves as similarly self-contained wholes. To be validated, then, one has to allow room for others and thereby concede one's lack of self-containment. Conjugal partners realize that the price of satisfying their selfish, bodily desires is a commitment to the other partner, making devotion, discipline and work more paramount in their lives than pleasure. When sincere, love involves a sense of loss. Partners give each other presents as externalization of that sense. Throughout all organizational units, from the couple to the state, the pattern repeats. Couples wishing for social recognition have to go through the elaborate marriage rites not because these rites directly express their feelings for each other, but because they do not: these rites are instead signs of obedience to a social whole which is larger than the couple. In the ultimate unit, one willingly offers to sacrifice everything. The unit that can legitimately ask for such a willingness has no other, bigger unit to merge into. It is the arms-bearing, troop-mobilizing and convict-executing sovereign state. Its relationship with other states is conflictual and warlike because there is no mediator beyond them. The internally split but ultimately unified self Fairbairn describes reflects Hegel's view of mind as universally single while still being divided against itself in each particular setting. Fairbairn's description of the self's itinerary towards integration as a process that involves acknowledging one's limits echoes Hegel's dialectic. Fairbairn's perception of civic participation, along with its discomforts and risks, as indicating personal integration, is similarly Hegelian. Fairbairn does not expect politics and civic bodies to be kind or provide deep gratification. Fairbairn (1952: 78–79, 239–244) does view them as unique forms of participation that acknowledge the scope of personal integration. Politics occurs among such mature actors and may involve risking their lives.

Things are different for Winnicott. The difference, however, is not a polar opposition. If Winnicott does not openly declare it, his description of the psychic trajectory in childhood is markedly Hegelian, as noted by Benjamin (1999: 191–192). In Winnicott, the child differentiates from the mother by destroying her, witnessing her survival of that destruction and then engaging with her as another human. By experiencing the deflection of one's destructive wishes as emanating from another human who is independent from the self, that self can be reconciled to its own relativity, and paradoxically to its own wholeness as another subject. So far, this account looks dialectic, and could have been expected to replicate elsewhere: by simply extending it, Winnicott would have been left with a worldview in which conflict is the price of authenticity. However, by introducing transitional space and the play activities based on it, Winnicott installs a bypass into the dialectic and neutralizes the function that conflict plays within it. Instead of making all subsequent recognition of peers and partners conditional on an existential struggle, the experience of mobilizing the mother's absence into the empowering and comforting transitional object assures that subsequent differences are met with curiosity and confidence rather than primarily with anxiety and aggression. 'In the experience of the more fortunate baby', Winnicott (1991: 108–109) writes, 'the question of separation…does not arise, because in the potential space between the baby and the mother there appears the creative playing that arises naturally out of the relaxed state'. Ian Suttie's endogenous repression is thereby given a more structured theoretical footing than Suttie himself had provided. The persistence of conflict that blights Hegel's and Fairbairn's world does not materialize in Winnicott.

This does not mean that Winnicott is a simplistically naïve anarchist. As Alford (2019: 51–56) notes, Winnicott is not a utopian thinker, for at least two reasons. The first is the retention of Klein's model at his background.

That model allows for reparation and concern, but nonetheless posits an irreducible layer of fear and aggression. By endorsing Klein, Winnicott endorses the perpetually agonistic hue of her worldview. The second reason is that Winnicott's basis in paediatric observation induces a recognition of children's ruthless aggression as an expression of physiological growth. Very early on, we experience violence both as an assertion of the self on the physical level and as necessary for protecting the self on the internal, psychic one. Taken together, these two factors install a measure of conflict into Winnicott's view of health. To this account, one should add a third reason for Winnicott's avoidance of utopia. Individual maturation is a complex process that experiences inevitable failures. If integration is a difficult task for individuals, it is even more so for an entire society, where the unhealthy members test the resilience of the rest. Between different societies that are separated by borders and jurisdiction, tensions are even greater. If just one actor turns aggressive due to an underlying pressure or illness, the others have to do so too for their own survival. 'Peace', Winnicott (1986: 212) warns, 'is very difficult to maintain…for more than a certain number of years'. Violence is constantly on the horizon of societal life (219).

The necessity of politics and states is a consequence of how precarious the achievement of individual health is. The existence of empowered public bodies is essential for managing politics. Winnicott dismisses attempts to construct a world government that would eventually engulf the familiar national constitutions and arbitrate their conflicts. The utopian desire to dispense with national differences and territorial borders, Winnicott (1986: 226–227, 256) thinks, expresses the very intolerance it strives to stamp out, channelling a denial of inner complexity. Winnicott thus retains both the unmediated, decisional potential of public life, and the institutions meant to process and regulate it. Unlike Hanna Arendt, Winnicott does not anticipate that smaller, more accessible forums will substitute elected magistracies and representative assemblies (Lederman, 2014: 332–333; McIvor, 2017). The reality of force-wielding institutions hardly matches with the rationale of the holding relationship. Winnicott can accordingly absolve himself from the suspicion of subsuming all meaningful adult activities under the transitional, intersubjective and creative title of play.

However, as LeJeune (2017) observes, precisely because Winnicott is aware that the peacefulness of the home cannot wholly supplant the unmediated contest of public, political life, he emphasizes the role of other, non-political activities that accumulate into culture. If healthy development hinges upon transitional space and the ability to play, then it assumes the individual's ability to invest a part of external reality with a personal meaning that is respected and reacted upon by the environment. Play instils a sense of agency and creativity through the very experience of resistance: play is enjoyable precisely because we cannot determine or anticipate our play-partner's moves. As play is externalized and socialized rather than merely fantasied, it links individuality to society as well as to physical reality. Consequentially, the friction and resistance met with in later life are not necessarily experienced as sacrifice to the alien objectivity of things. Instead, we cherish them as part of an empowering and bonding life. Through play, Winnicott (1988: 111) writes, 'feeling remains that the world is personally created'. It is our world: we need not offer our lives as a sign of recognizing its alterity. Culture, religion, art, sports and science are all based on play. They cover large swaths of social experience, making most of it potentially rewarding without a price to be paid in impersonality, pain, conflict and death.

The various levels of integration and attachment enabled by play and culture are neither mutually exclusive nor confined by territorial boundaries. Democracies attuned towards their healthy members foster the elaboration of culture and its multiple occasions. Their scope can be as narrow as the local club and as wide as the world. The sites where they unfold need not be mutually exclusive. If Winnicott discards the idea of world citizenship in the technical sense of all humans holding identity cards issued by the same state, he nonetheless views awareness of humanity's shared universe as a viable, if relatively rare, sign of health:

> [T]he unit personality is part of a wider concept of wholeness. And soon will be part of a social life of an ever-widening kind; and of political matters and...of something that can be called world-citizenship. (1986: 60)

Even short of such identification with humanity as a whole, attachment to culture renders its participants reluctant to use violence. While they can be convinced of war's inevitability, they are slow to accept it, as the logic of war negates the cooperative quality of culture. If the web of cultural sites cannot enforce peace, its many participants may postpone and diminish war through their tendency to 'miss the bus to the front line' (Winnicott, 1986: 258).

The politics of governments, borders and wars may be increasingly domesticated by a culture that grows out of the initial bond, which is at the same time the hub of the private sphere and the first holder of rights against external intervention. The role of politics becomes subsidiary rather than substantial: it covers up for the places where healthy development has not taken place, rather than providing a channel for healthy development to prove itself, as in Hegel and Fairbairn. Pure destruction is unleashed once, when the child attacks the mother. After she survives and is established as a real person, destruction turns to the symbolic rivalry of play and derivative activities. Aggression, and therefore risk and the possibility of sacrifice have no essential role.

Avoiding Decision

The near-absence in Winnicott's scheme of politics as an independent sphere has troubled scholars. Overall supportive of Winnicott's stand on mind and society, Flax (1993a: 45) cautions that the sphere of decision and force should not be reduced to the terms of the first relationship. The context of citizenship, politics and law is radically different from that of the home and the parent-child bond. It follows that a distinct, unique sphere of politics should be the corollary of the healthy home Winnicott describes, not as a regrettable necessity, but as a logical counterpart that arises from our understanding of where the vulnerability of childhood and primary relationships should be respected.

Would the outcome not be a civic sphere that is wholly alien to the intimacy of the home, friendship and culture? Flax (1993b) responds that such a stark opposition is not essential. Winnicott's view of individual differentiation as synergetic with reciprocal recognition may still inform our concepts of justice and citizenship. These supposedly public spaces may stand for an intermediate plane between self and other rather than consist in an elevated viewpoint external to both. How, then, can Winnicott both concede the contributory role of a distinct civic realm and relate it to his psychological model so as to enrich public life? One way to answer this is to view Winnicott as capable of addressing dilemmas that political philosophers have been pondering for centuries. By contrasting the state to nature, early-modern authors, such as Hobbes, Locke and Rousseau, conceded that government was artificial. Nomos was not physis. Choosing to obey nomos involved a mental leap, an acceptance of a contrivance as a legitimate authority, which led to various problems in these classical formulations: why should we commit to a sovereign whom we know to be fictional? If we do obey the sovereign, do we not negate our inner nature? If we do not obey, do we not doom ourselves to a stagnant, animal-like existence? Winnicott shows a way out of this conundrum. The adults respect the child's view of the teddy and the child accepts the rules of the game because such respect is necessary for meaningful communication to unfold, and that communication is their most authentic and persistent wish. Positive legislation and civic discipline could in principle be considered such transitional phenomena as well, rendering them crucial for a culture made of creative and confident individuals.

Following on that, Winnicott could also provide the therapeutic rationale and motivation for endorsing the element of ultimate obligation and potential sacrifice involved in politics. To create transitional space, both a sense of internal depth and a recognition of outer reality are required. The sense of a hard objectivity that does not yield, a platform of solid rock that cannot be moulded by our feet, is accordingly a condition of health. Like the biting and pushing child, we look for an outer boundary to resist us. However, constantly courting hardship and risk is hardly compatible with everyday life. Instead, the necessary outer boundary could be furnished by a commitment to a final ruling that originates from outside each individual. In a secular world, such decisions may only originate in other humans. If one proceeds from egalitarian, liberal and democratic premises, these other humans have to be a constitutional majority. The availability of politics as an arena where one engages with other citizens to formulate a final, obligating decision could therefore be framed in Winnicott's terms as concomitant of health. The artificial nature of such a commitment should not overly concern us if we accept the dynamics of transition and play.

The notion of a committing civic life as therapeutic does appear in some political tracts. Liberal thinkers like Benjamin Constant, and, to a certain degree, J.S. Mill, saw the involvement with political bodies and civic duties, difficult and dangerous though it may be, as a remedial counterweight to the chaotic fluidity of internal life. Medieval civilization rested on the imaginative precepts of heaven and hell; the civic politics of enlightenment, by contrast, rested on real other people. Constitutional democracy was preferable to medieval autocracy not because it was more rational or just, but because it could take us outside our volatile imagination (Manent, 1995; Rosenblum, 1987). We respect majoritarian decision and constitutional law as imperatives, because, unlike theology and myth, civic politics involves other people who are real to us rather than representations of internal forces that evoke visceral responses from us. A world tormented by the opposing claims that differing religions made on their believers' internal lives could be rescued by investing itself in the intersubjective space offered by the state. Hobbes, to take some liberty with Bill Watterson's popular comic strip, became Calvin's transitional object.

Nonetheless, if these are all possible readings of Winnicott's theory, then they are unlikely to be approved by Winnicott himself. The operation of governments, states and armed forces involves lethal violence and necessitates irreversible decisions. Such a necessity is not part of transitional space and does not appear in play as Winnicott understands it: in play, responsibility is limited. Transitional space, Winnicott (1988: 107) writes, is a place where subjectivity and objectivity meet but do not conflict: within it the child 'does not have to decide'. With transition, the remnants of the fantasied struggle between infant and mother that Winnicott had inherited from Klein are resolved: the self and the other can safely recognize both their differences and their connection. On the shoreline, one can inhabit land and sea at the same time. As transition permeates the subsequent lives of healthy individuals, existential choices take a back seat in their experiences. The need for a public discussion of such choices similarly declines in the society these individuals coalesce into. They do not view its public affairs as anxiety-generating, urgent ones. Winnicott (1986: 233) argues that one outcome of health is a naïve trust in shared social reality, a consequence of a reassuring early holding. Such confidence distances the healthy and integrated individuals from engagement with politics, thus rendering them vulnerable to the machinations of the sick, who dabble in politics as a venue for their desire to dominate and control. Politics remains a regrettable, but progressively less urgent necessity, rather than an occasion for engagement, a fading blemish on the otherwise peaceful, if imperfect, world of transition and play.

Winnicott's rejection of utopia leaves him safely within the liberal camp, as does his focus on individual creativity and the need to respect private sites. But his expectation that play-based activities will progressively, if never completely, diminish the impact of politics indicates that he expects the civic realm to gradually, if never perfectly, shed its distinctness. This perception distances Winnicott from the classical, veteran liberalism of Locke and Mill. As the holding relationship Winnicott envisions is not simply static but instead generates the dynamic capacity for play and creativity, his model anticipates the perpetual growth of the private realm based on play and creativity. The liberty he wishes to protect is both a universal, and therefore categorically obliging, space, and a springboard for each person to formulate and pursue their own ends. As that space is natural and hallowed, criticism of its internal divisions becomes irrelevant: such criticism draws its terms from the conflicted, and not wholly substantial, realm of politics. Parenting roles and gender essences are placed beyond scrutiny, while the civic sphere and its organs are understood as a declining instrument of the peaceful and dynamic private sphere.

References

Alexander, S. (2012). Primary maternal preoccupation: D.W. Winnicott and social democracy in mid-twentieth-century Britain. In Alexander, S., and Taylor, B. (eds.), *History and psyche: Culture, psychoanalysis, and the past.* New York: Palgrave, 149–172.

Alford, C.F. (2000). Levinas and Winnicott: Motherhood and responsibility. *American Imago* 57 (3): 235–239.

Alford, C.F. (2019). Hate, aggression, and recognition. In Allen, A., and O'Connor, B. (eds.), *Transitional subjects: Critical theory and object relations.* New York: Columbia University Press, 51–73.

Benjamin, J. (1999). Recognition and destruction: An outline of intersubjectivity. In Mitchell, S.A., and Aron, L. (eds.), *Relational psychoanalysis: The emergence of a tradition.* Hillsdale, NJ: The Analytic Press, 181–210.

Doane, J., and Hodges, D. (1992). *From Klein to Kristeva.* Ann Arbor: University of Michigan Press.

Eyer, D. (1992). *Mother-Infant bonding.* New Haven, CT: Yale University Press.

Fairbairn, W.R.D. (1952). *Psychoanalytic studies of the personality.* London: Routledge and Kegan Paul.

Flax, J. (1990). *Thinking fragments.* Berkeley and Los Angeles: University of California Press.

Flax, J. (1993a). *Disputed subjects*. London and New York: Routledge.
Flax, J. (1993b). The play of justice: Justice as a transitional space. *Political Psychology* 15: 331–346.
Gerson, G. (2005). Individuality, deliberation and welfare in Donald Winnicott. *History of the Human Sciences* 18 (1): 107–126.
Gerson, G. (2017). Winnicott and the history of welfare state thought in Britain. In Bowker, M.H., and Buzby, A. (eds.), *D.W. Winnicott and political theory*. New York: Palgrave, 311–332.
Greenberg, J.R., and Mitchell, S.A. (1983). *Object relations in psychoanalytic theory*. Cambridge, MA: Harvard University Press.
Hegel, G.W.F. (1952). *Hegel's philosophy of right*. Ed. T.M. Knox. Oxford: Clarendon.
Hoggett, P. (1992). *Partisans in an uncertain world: The psychoanalysis of engagement*. London: Free Association.
Jacobs, M. (1988). *D.W. Winnicott*. London: Sage.
Kahr, B. (1996). *D.W. Winnicott: A biographical portrait*. London: Karnac Books.
Lederman, S. (2014). Agonism and deliberation in Arendt. *Constellations* 21 (3): 327–337.
LeJeune, J. (2017). Adults in the playground: Winnicott and Arendt on politics and playfulness. In Bowker, M., and Buzby, A. (eds.), *D.W. Winnicott and political theory*. New York: Palgrave, 247–268.
Locke, J. (1946). *The second treatise of civil government*. Oxford: Basil Blackwell.
Manent, P. (1995). *An intellectual history of liberalism*. Princeton, NJ: Princeton University Press.
McIvor, D. (2017). In transition, but to where? Winnicott, integration, and democratic associations. In Bowker, M., and Buzby, A. (eds.), *D.W. Winnicott and political theory*. New York: Palgrave, 205–227.
Mill, J.S. (1977). *The collected works of John Stuart Mill*, Vol. XVIII. Ed. J.M. Robson. Toronto: University of Toronto Press.
Minsky, M. (1996). *Psychoanalysis and gender*. New York and London: Routledge.
Nussbaum, M. (2006). Winnicott on the surprises of the self. *The Massachusetts Review* 47 (2): 375–393.
Phillips, A. (1989). *Winnicott*. Cambridge, MA: Harvard University Press.
Riley, D. (1983). *War in the nursery*. London: Virago.
Rodman, F.R. (2003). *Winnicott*. Cambridge, MA: Perseus.
Rosenblum, N.L. (1987). *Another liberalism*. Cambridge, MA: Harvard University Press.
Rudnytsky, P.L. (2002). *Reading psychoanalysis*. Ithaca, NY and London: Cornell University Press.
Rustin, M. (1991). *The good society and the inner world*. London and New York: Verso.
Scharff, D.E. (2005). The development of Fairbairn's theory. In Scharff, J.S., and Scharff, D.E. (eds.), *The legacy of Fairbairn and Sutherland*. London and New York: Routledge, 3–18.
Shapira, M. (2013). *The war inside*. Cambridge: Cambridge University Press.
Winnicott, D.W. (1950). *The ordinary devoted mother and her baby*. London: private edition.
Winnicott, D.W. (1965a). *The family and individual development*. London: Tavistock.

Winnicott, D.W. (1965b). *The maturational processes and the facilitating environment.* London: Hogarth.
Winnicott, D.W. (1971). *Therapeutic consultations in child psychiatry.* London: Hogarth.
Winnicott, D.W. (1975). *Through paediatrics to psycho-analysis.* London: Hogarth.
Winnicott, D.W. (1984). *Through paediatrics to psychoanalysis.* London: Karnac.
Winnicott, D.W. (1986). *Home is where we start from.* New York and London: W.W. Norton.
Winnicott, D.W. (1988). *Human nature.* London: Free Association.
Winnicott, D.W. (1989) *Holding and Interpretation.* London: Karnac.
Winnicott, D.W. (1991). *Playing and reality.* London and New York: Routledge.

5 Play in the Open Society

Winnicott and Popper

This chapter points to the similarities between some of Winnicott's ideas, on the one hand, and those of Karl Popper, the philosopher of science who was roughly Winnicott's coeval, on the other hand. Initially, Popper and Winnicott seem to have scant common ground. Popper (2002: 34–37) criticized psychoanalysis for failing, as he saw it, the test of falsification by which science is known. Despite this, however, reading their works side by side can highlight the places where object relations thought coalesced with a broader ideological trend than British liberal philosophy's realignment towards the welfare state. That realignment itself concurred with the increasing preponderance of a wider, Atlantic ideology that perceived human liberty as unfolding in more than the framework of the national, territorial state: freedom was now a universal entitlement that exceeded electorates and borders and could manifest in countless ways and activities, a character of a rich and diverse civilization rather than of formal citizenship. Popper summarized this approach with the phrase 'the open society'. Winnicott and through him object relations thought taken as a whole are compatible with this vision.

Psychology as a Holistic Worldview

Object relations theory's tendency to normatively and descriptively bypass politics is fundamental. The very contents of object relations theory render it a theory of a unified realm where essential splits between privacy and publicity, individual and social, feature mainly as errors and disruptions. Freud's own intervention already questioned the distinction between individual psychology, on the one hand, and disciplines such as sociology and political philosophy, on the other hand. All social units, including the largest ones, could be examined through the psychoanalytical lens, shedding doubt on the justifications and explanations previously offered to make sense of them. Endorsing psychoanalysis, some critics feared, would jeopardize any ability to perceive a shared, common arena which exceeds private desire, leading to the substitution of political ideals by an inward-looking, and ultimately futile, cultivation of the self (Nachman, 1981; Rieff, 1966).

However, classical psychoanalysis also resists its extension to political theory, for at least two reasons. The first is Freud's caution. Freud is often castigated as a nineteenth-century positivist who imposed the vocabulary of mechanic pressures on the mind's subtler and more organic workings. But the same positivism meant that Freud saw psychoanalysis as a form of guesswork called for in the absence of direct access to brain processes (Wallace, 1992). His theory was a second-best, a provisional aid required where crisper data are unavailable. If social and political conclusions followed from psychoanalysis, they acquired the same heuristic character, thus avoiding an authoritative pronouncement on society and its institutions. Consequently, even in his metapsychological essays, Freud mainly tells his audience what not to do. He has almost no positive recommendations. The second reason for classical psychoanalysis's evasion of a too-ready conversion into social thought has to do with its contents. Freud's account of the mind involves a series of transformative shocks, leading to the repression of entire classes of experiences. Our lives are always split between conscious and unconscious. Our being is inevitably divided against itself. Any assertion of homogeneity is a defence against that division, and so extracts its inevitable prices. The Christian love preached by the clergy holds within the denominational community, but becomes genocidal hatred in proportion to its emotional intensity when one ventures outside that community: one set of rules applies in one location, a completely different one in the next. There is no generalized guideline that can apply to us both as separate individuals and as members of a group. Based on its classical, Viennese phase, then, psychoanalytic knowledge views itself as limited and partial. It describes a discontinuity between organizational levels which further discourages the extension of individual psychology to society at large.

In object relations theory, by comparison, both these impediments are weaker. Inspired by Freud's therapeutic talking-cure method more than by his theory, object relations authors from Ian Suttie on understood communication as the key to healing. Communication takes place with another human and its contents are specific to that human. Subjectivity is thus a valid source of understanding rather than a distorted reflection of objectivity. The ideal reference point is no longer a wholly objective scheme with its predictable repetitions as in physical science. It is, instead, an understanding that includes a dialogic and interpretive dimension: knowledge about humans originates in humans and their experiences. Unlike Freud, then, object relations theorists could dispense with the notion of psychoanalysis as a provisional, flawed substitute for science. Psychoanalysis could become a source of understanding on par with the exact sciences. Relations-based psychoanalysis could accordingly stake out more comprehensive statements about individuals and society alike. Extending the insights of object relations theory from the individual patient and the early home environment to civilization at large was less of a metapsychological stretch than it had been for Freud. Additionally, the contents of object relations theory do not primarily deal with inevitable traumatic breaks as in classical analysis. Instead, object relations thought focuses on the unfolding of the relating self's characters and capabilities, and on the many forms the self's attachment to its environment take. Nothing human is placed beyond the fundamental template of relating. Object relations theory, then, envisages an integrated, if differentiated, field for its enquiry. Politics and civic activities are not held apart from other pursuits. They are different expressions of the same underlying, integrated realm.

For the same reason, object relations theory is inhospitable to notions of an essential or even merely methodological divide between psyche and society. For Freud, illness primarily manifested as difficulty in keeping private, internal contents away from publicly visible functioning. The patient zero of classical psychoanalysis was a hysteric: the woman whose functioning was impaired by a repressed internal struggle to the point where that struggle showed as a somatic and motoric handicap. Therapy was about rearranging the psychic contents and restoring the public, functioning persona. By contrast, the patient zero of object relations analysis is a schizoid, a person whose external behaviour may look ordinary at first but is nonetheless found on additional examination to be constantly eroded by its divorce from internal motivation. The schizoid patients whom Fairbairn (1952: 84–85) saw in his Edinburgh clinic in the 1930s alerted him to the blind spots of classical analysis. By partitioning their emotional lives from their acting personas, these patients acquired the ability to go through the motions of Freudian treatment without being genuinely touched by it, pressuring the therapist for changing his approach and consequently triggering the theoretical shift from physical drive to relating. If relating was the main motivation, then the division of external functioning alongside others from an internal wish to engage in and be rewarded by such functioning stood as the paradigmatic illness. The fundamental psychotherapeutic problem, Fairbairn thought, was not an innate destructive urge. It was, instead, the internal splitting of communicative from non-communicative parts of the personality. Rather than a hostile, paranoid stance towards the world, 'the basic position in the psyche is invariably a schizoid position' (8). But as object relations theory was still psychoanalysis, such splitting did not necessarily present itself in a declared, consciously alienated or rebellious form. It operated surreptitiously through the distancing between emotion and conduct, privacy and publicness. In the form of the false self, the schizoid phenomenon remained a preoccupation for Winnicott as it had been for Fairbairn. Guntrip (2001: 238), who drew inspiration from both Fairbairn and Winnicott, declared that for object relations psychoanalysis, 'the schizoid problem…*is* the *ultimate problem*'. The statement applied not just to emotions and conduct, but also to cognition, as in the pedantic distancing of hard science from feelings or in the legalist insistence on one's rights as detached from any ethical obligation. The moral and civilizational implications of schizoid phenomena were further registered by R.D. Laing's phrase 'the divided self' and the popularity the notion gained in broader culture (Laing, 1965). From a position informed by object relations theory, the division of public and private was a manifestation of disorder that ripped through the enriching, benign and dynamic forms that interpersonal dialogue could take. Advocating the autonomy of politics from other concerns was one of its variants.

Democracy's Future at the Midcentury

This refusal to detach politics as a subject from the more comprehensive, humanistic notion of knowledge and reason echoes the midcentury's reformulation of liberalism and democracy. The unsettling experiences of the World Wars and their aftermath indicated to many that the West's democracy was not facing a single ideological rival, but several, and that their common denominator was their empowerment of political bodies. Totalitarianism could be left or right, but it always made the state unique and supreme by arguing that it could do things that other bodies could not do, and that its actions could not be assessed by standards taken from other fields. As against this, democracy began to think of itself not just as a form of government, but as a civilization of which government was a branch and a servant. The veteran liberal notion of placing limits on the state found a footing in this perception.

The advanced liberalism of the welfare state concurred with this turn. For many of the welfare state's liberal advocates, tasking government with furnishing suitable economic and social conditions for its citizens was a particle of a broader vision. It included a transition from a world of competing interests, rival ideologies and warring states to a more peaceful civilization characterized by constantly diversifying contacts and modes of cooperation among individuals and the associations they form, transcending their civic loyalties. Placing such a vision on the horizon of the welfare state project was necessary for justifying the expansion of governmental functions to include matters like the education and health of individuals in their everyday lives. If the significance of government lowered because additional human bonds created more societal sites and institutions, then government could be entrusted with a broader mandate without incurring the fear that its power might expand correspondingly. Developing bonds were expected to be driven by the accumulating choices of their individual participants and were not necessarily expressed through formally political institutions. Individual citizens' freedom to create such ties was to be assured by political institutions, but the products of this freedom did not end up by strengthening such institutions. Protected by welfare rights, individuals could venture into activities and affiliations where their aspirations played out within egalitarian, voluntarily chosen environments. These environments accumulated into a worldwide civilization (Rosenboim, 2017).

As argued earlier, the philosophical basis for this expectation was created by synthesizing several sources of liberal thought. Chiefly, Locke's perception of a natural society that underlies all legitimate institutions combined with Mill's idea of liberty as individual self-realization. A natural, and therefore universal, society always existed beneath all visible offices and magistracies. Its products were confident and free actors who engaged in ever-developing ventures. As a secondary institution that had to appeal to the underlying natural society for legitimation, the state was merely a technical enabler, and was committed to respecting the evolving choices of individuals if it was to maintain its legitimacy. As a result, the politics of parliaments and governments could be understood as a provisional go-between that enabled the growth of an enfolding, universally human web of activities and associations that was identical to the idea of a free society. Issued in 1941 as a statement of war aims by the Western allies, the Atlantic Charter numbered welfare alongside the individual rights to life and liberty as components of a projected peaceful order. The welfare state was to become a constituent of a larger world that operated along liberal and democratic principles. Beveridge, the author most commonly associated with the British welfare state programme, expected peace to be achieved on the basis of non-sovereign democracies committed to the liberty and well-being of their citizens and to humans everywhere (Beveridge, 1945: 51–52). For such a settlement to hold, Beveridge (1940) thought, the often-opposing of its constituents-armed governments-had to be tempered by cultivating ties between populations, so that they would form into a global society that would coexist with, but would not be equivalent to, the alliances contracted into by governments. Science, trade and culture were to flank institutional politics.

Comparable ideas were endorsed at the time by some of welfare liberalism's ideological rivals on right and left. An outline comparable to this vision was proposed, for example, by Friedrich Hayek, from premises that seemed to unambiguously reject welfare liberalism by assuming that enlarging government to deal with citizens' living conditions would undermine rather than bolster individual liberty. Hayek suspected that the expansion of governmental agencies involved in the welfare project constituted the first step towards an authoritarian regime from the clutches of which there would be no return. With bureaucracies assuming additional responsibilities and the populace becoming dependent on them, democratic leverage and individual liberties would decline to a critical point beyond which the process would be irreversible. For the economic planning necessitated by the welfare state, Hayek substituted the free market as a fair, neutral and efficient mediator. Hayek's trust in the market spilled over into his view of international relations, war and peace, and the projected future organization of the entire world. But, paradoxically, this approach landed him in a position not very far from Beveridge's as it included the anticipation of a global society that would tame power politics, conflict and war by enfolding expressly political, coercive institutions within other ties and bonds, consequently reducing the relative impact of political bodies. While suggesting a formal international mechanism to delay and possibly avert future war, Hayek (2007, 2011) also hoped that the growing ties propelled by the expansion of trade would create a universally public, but not political or civic, arena, whose operation would overshadow the formal politics of states and diminish their preoccupation with enforcement and conflict.

On the welfare-oriented liberals' left, Harold Laski formulated a socialist and pluralist agenda that avoided, as he saw it, the centralization and bureaucratization entailed by Beveridge's plan. Laski entrusted voluntary associations such as trade unions and municipal forums rather than governmental offices with enabling individuals to create bonds of solidarity. He contrasted the social landscape composed of such groups with the impersonality of government and the dehumanizing competition of the market alike. However, as these associations were voluntary, they ultimately depended on individual choice, and that choice was guaranteed as a constitutional right upheld by the governmental agencies responsible for shielding individuals from crime, external aggression and the many inequalities of the workplace and trade. As the groupings created by free individuals take normative priority over governmental edicts, they cannot be limited by borders and nationalities, and become global. These activities are all voluntary, entailing that the associations based on them are not oppressive and do not incur overwhelming tensions. As a result, Laski (1938, 1943) ends up by sharing Beveridge's and Hayek's anticipation of a world order where activities emanating from the private, formally and legally protected concerns of citizens spin a web of commitments and affiliations that can be expected to gradually temper the power play and polarized interests of governments, states and rulers (Lamb, 2004: 147–173). A civilization of autonomous but interacting agents enfolds and eventually overshadows politics as conventionally perceived.

Ideas related to this notion of a worldwide free society were elaborated by authors arguing, not only from differing ideological bases, but from within various professions and disciplines. Scholars of international relations voiced their versions of this agenda, as did activists interested in resolving the problems of employment and industrial organization (Carr, 1945; Holthaus, 2014; Mitrany, 1943). Whether understood as a sphere where individuals pursue their own interests while being protected by welfare rights, as a realm for trade and economic initiative, or as an area inhabited by communities and groups, the private realm was expected by these many authors to influence, if never obviate, the behaviour of states and formal civic bodies. In all cases, the anticipation was that individual liberty would be guaranteed by government, taking the form of juristic entitlement. The exchanges and relationships generated by individuals enjoying this freedom were to extend out of the original shielded bubble of welfare, free trade or voluntary association, and form a multilayered universal community in which government's significance would be relatively weakened.

Dialogue, Knowledge and Freedom

Few individuals were more axial than Karl Popper was in advancing the perception of liberal democracy as geared to foster a civilization in which political bodies take a subsidiary role to the contacts and practices that free-choosing individuals create. Popper saw political institutions as necessary but regrettable hindrances to a conversation that occurs among free individuals. Granting political institutions and the activities that occur around them any special status meant suppressing that conversation. Hence, a free society was one in which politics was subsidiary to dialogue.

Aiming at a common ground for the various legitimations of democracy, Popper (1966, v. 1) offered the concept of the open society as their shared hub. Elaborated and presented towards the end of the Second World War, the concept accommodated perspectives as far apart as those of Hayek and Laski, whom Popper regarded as ideological allies despite their apparent polarity (Hacohen, 2000: 449). When propelling his approach, Popper succeeded to the degree of having the idea of the open society widely accepted into the terminology of the post-war world and becoming nearly synonymous with Western democracy itself (Hacohen, 2000: 449, 557; Stokes, 1998: 72).

For Popper, totalitarian regimes of all ideological stripes are variants on what he calls the closed society, a civilization that adheres to a single, inalterable account that encompasses all knowledge. The closed society confronts its residents with a world that cannot be challenged, of which their own lives are but manifestations. This is characteristic of isolated and archaic societies as it is of modern totalitarianism. Closed-society thought relegates power to agents who claim to embody the dominant system of knowledge. The social hierarchy thus grounded declares itself an inflection of a given universe. Both personal leverage and political liberty are suppressed. The closed society's manifestations in Western history are sophisticated, as they have been transmitted through refined and tightly argued philosophies. These provided the groundwork for ancient tyranny as they shored up twentieth-century totalitarianism. Popper numbers Plato; Aristotle; Hegel; Marx; and, to a lesser degree, Freud as purveyors of closed-society thought. Their theories require that we accept their revelatory statements about ideal forms, teleology, spiritual and material dialectic, and the unconscious. Disbelief is condemned as moral, intellectual or medical failure (Popper 1966 v. 1: 57–73).

By contrast, democracy proceeds from doubt and the readiness to listen, explore and innovate. Democratic government does not stand for a single and final truth but instead registers the often conflicting positions of its many participants. This does not mean that democracy is devoid of philosophical coherence. A thorough Kantian, Popper believes in a truth-out-there as he believes in its inaccessibility to the senses. Popper suggests that the mediation between humans' flawed subjectivity and the objective world takes place through engagement among subjectivities. Such engagements occur on a continuous, practical, everyday basis, manifesting how essential they are to humans. Popper continues here from the work of the Austrian school of economic thought. The school's authors suggested that trade bridges individual players' beliefs with the given pressures of the economy. An item's price reflects both the objectively measurable quantities of work and material invested in its production, and the subjectively grounded expectations that sellers and buyers entertain. None of these qualities exhausts the good's real value, but their interplay, as expressed in the price paid, is as good a reflection as possible of that value. While factoring in both measurable fact and sensed experience, the price is distinct from both (Hacohen, 2000: 465–469).

Popper suggests that, alongside the market, an entire class of phenomena exist that are produced by inputs from separate individuals, but display themselves to each person as independent from their felt wishes. Language is not strictly an out-there, objectively existing item. The use of a noun to denote a thing is not one of that thing's immutable properties. It is an ultimately random representation of that item and has no life outside that given to it by the speakers. But the speakers still accept grammatical and pronunciation principles rather than invent them. Each speaker treats a phenomenon that exists only through other speakers' subjectivities as if it were an obliging facet of a given world. Exclusively rooted neither in speakers' musings nor in unnegotiable materiality, market and language are members of what Popper calls the third world, that space that lies beyond the world of facts and that of sensations, while connecting these two worlds and evolving its own internal rules (Popper, 1979: 106–107).

Third-world phenomena help us to act realistically by giving room to subjectivity. Our perceptions are coloured by our circumstances and are therefore inaccurate measures of reality. But they are not completely illusory: related, in however complex a way, to inputs from reality, perceptions are partial but valid. By respecting and giving attention to others' (admittedly skewed) perceptions as they respect and give attention to ours, we can collectively improve our understanding of reality. From this process of mutual examination, provisional agreement gradually emerges.

Endorsing it, participants modify their own perceptions and therefore have new inputs to offer, propelling the discussion onwards. A third-world phenomenon arises when such a conversation is enabled, constituting a field of knowledge made by subjective statements but advancing towards a better account of objective reality. This is the basis of scholarly disciplines and can be equated with science itself. The 'inter-subjectivity of scientific method', Popper (1966 v. 2: 217) writes, provides humans with workable knowledge and collective progress.

Third-world engagements depend on the equality and liberty of their participants. Discussion is derailed and its contents depleted if contributions are rejected because of their authors' identity and status rather than because of their contents. Every person should be treated as a potential contributor and every opinion should be debatable. Correspondingly, every participant concedes that their own dearly held beliefs can be criticized and demolished, creating legitimate space for others to express their opinion, and committing themselves to the proviso '*I may be wrong and you may be right*' (Popper, 1966 v. 2: 225). Just as any person's account is fallible, so are the conclusions reached collectively through conversation. Challenges to them should be heard as well, so as to avoid the termination of the debate and the creation of an unnegotiable final truth. To avoid such closure, participants in open and egalitarian conversation treat even beliefs made consensual by their own debate as provisional and awaiting disproof (Hacohen, 2000: 513; Shearmur, 1996: 81–82).

A society geared for cultivating third-world conversations counts each person as the next, allows different opinions and outlooks to form and be expressed, avoids a final, unchangeable verdict, and proceeds by rules that apply equally to all and are known by all. It is an open society. Its political form is constitutional democracy (Popper, 1966 v. 1: 1–3). Whatever its other specifications, democracy guarantees constitutional rights so that individuals can make their own choices, broadcast their opinions, and be accessible to inputs from others.

Life in the open society, Popper (1966 v. 1: 70–73) admits, is beset by uncertainty and controversy. Its constituents are burdened by the realization that no knowledge and no social arrangement can be perfect, and that no certainty about the value of one's actions can be had. Popper nonetheless expects the open society to prevail over the alternative. Within the closed society, innovation and exploration are stifled. Its individual constituents are particles who have predetermined parts to perform within a whole rather than wholes who can hold their own perceptions. By contrast, the open society guarantees individual entitlements and so assures conditions for new ideas and better solutions to emerge, rendering it stronger in the long term. The room for innovation gained by dialogue between freely expressed thoughts and ideas assures the durability of the collective as well as generating space for the individuals' use and discretion (Popper, 2008: 313–328, 388–390).

Play as Freedom

This notion of freedom and movement as rooted in the meeting of mutually recognizing subjects is crucial for Winnicott's outlook as it is for Popper's. For Winnicott, the play activities that develop from within conditions of secure holding establish a sense of individual agency. This is itself a private case of a broader principle in Winnicott. Healthy being is simultaneously internal and external, as excluding any of the two facets either locks the self in a claustrophobic and dead inside or forces the self to survive in an entirely alien environment. From the first stages of life and onwards, health associates with the ability to engage in gradual, limited-liability interactions with the environment. The child, Winnicott (1988: 129) writes, 'becomes accustomed to interruptions of continuity and begins to become able to allow for them provided they are not too severe or too prolonged'. The capacity to continue such challenging but regulated interactions with the world throughout life hinges around the child's act of recognizing the mother as existing beyond his or her omnipotent control. The mother becomes another person.

When the mother is perceived as another person rather than an engulfing environment or an internal part-object, the child gains the confidence and the elbow room to explore possibilities for movement and action through the patterns that become play. Rooted in engagement with transitional objects, play activities involve the investment of a given, concrete facet of reality with subjective feeling. The ability to play creates an opening between the shut-in interior and the alien, external world, standing for a 'variability…that is different in quality from the variabilities that belong to…psychic reality and to external or shared reality' (Winnicott, 1991: 107). Exceeding both subjectivity and objectivity, transition is the 'third part of…life' where change and growth take place (Winnicott, 1991: 2).

The interaction of child and mother furnishes the conditions of individual agency by providing it with motivation and channels. As playing involves manipulating objects that have volume and weight, it cultivates the skills of reflection, comparison and calibrating means to ends. It enables greater motoric agility and underlies the cognitive grasp over the physical world that precedes the development from magic to science (Winnicott, 1991: 11–12). Moreover, play allows actions that arise from within the self to be recognized and validated by others, thereby providing not just the space for exploration and creativity, but the emotional motivation for utilizing it. Rather than either fantasying or mechanically performing, one becomes a free human (Winnicott, 1991: 65–71). Play thus allows us to feel confident about our own reality as autonomous agents, while avoiding being overwhelmed by the acknowledgement that an objective alterity exists out there. We can concede both the partial, relative quality of our own subjectivity and the indifferent and limiting character of objectivity without falling apart (Winnicott, 1965: 148–150).

Social and political implications follow. One, generalized, implicit and largely negative implication is the avoidance of utopian visions that appeal to comprehensive and final knowledge. Transitional space and the rewarding play and play-like activities based on it deliver neither euphoric bliss nor flawless wisdom. The open-ended nature of individual agency – the sense that one can actually choose and make a change – generates discomforts that self-enclosed fantasying evades. Concern, guilt and the sadness that give the depressive position its name are the prices that one pays for the capacity to meaningfully act on one's own wishes and aspirations (Winnicott, 1991: 36). Agency's source in the recognition of the other as a subject like the self, moreover, includes the admission that others, too, are flawed and vulnerable rather than omnipotent and omniscient (Winnicott, 1991: 86–94). Knowledge of reality is transmitted and elaborated between such limited humans and is accordingly always partial. Accepting the conditions of individual freedom necessitates tolerating this provisional character of knowledge. 'I know', Winnicott (1988: 114–115) imagines the healthy individual as conceding, 'that there is no direct contact between external reality and myself, only an illusion of contact, a midway phenomenon that works very well for me'. Health renounces expectations of perfectibility.

The second, more positive and explicit consequence of identifying liberty with transitional space and transitional activities is a commitment to constitutional democracy. A polity geared for health should shield the home environment within which the twin processes of recognition and separation take place. That polity should be similarly invested in allowing individuals to externalize their autonomously developed wishes in settings that validate their creativity. Society's institutions and bodies should therefore stand away from the home while assuring an area free from interference for each individual (Winnicott, 1991: 109). Society, moreover, should see to it that individuals and homes are not hampered by other factors besides its own institutional arms. Poverty and economic insecurity are such factors. Constant worry about affording tuition fees or medical help, for example, can detract from the parent's ability to calmly hold the child. Families and individuals merit assistance from the collective (Winnicott, 1986: 246–249). The ensuing political structure is a liberal social-democracy that grants rights to individuals and families alike, while taking responsibility for the societal conditions of individual thriving by enacting education, health and welfare measures (Alexander, 2012; Hoggett, 2008; Rustin, 1991: 3–7, 150–152).

Popper and Winnicott, then, identify liberty with the meeting of one sentient and desiring but self-admittedly limited mind with others, who are acknowledged as similarly independent and flawed. For Popper, such encounters constitute third-world phenomena that release each person from the narrow horizons of received prejudices and mythologies, while advancing civilization by fostering workable knowledge. For Winnicott, transitional space frees children from encapsulation in fantasy while at the same time enabling them to accept the objective quality of the environment and, to a degree, impact that environment by externalizing content for response by others. Both authors derive from their concepts a political approach that upholds liberal democracy, discards utopian claims to social perfection and expects societal institutions to acknowledge the liberating force of the interpersonal meeting by guaranteeing the autonomy and safety of the sites where that meeting takes place.

Complementarity

Alongside the similarities their attitudes to the intersubjective plane and its liberating potential manifest, Popper and Winnicott are also capable of augmenting each other's outlooks. Popper's account raises two questions about the motivations required for engaging in the open society's dialogue. The first has to do with origins. The possibility of progress and liberty dawned, Popper thinks, in Greek Antiquity, when strangers began to compare their received beliefs. 'Telling their myth', he writes, 'they were ready in their turn to listen to what their listener thought about it – admitting thereby that he might have a better explanation' (Popper, 2002: 170). The arena was thus established in which one entrusts another person whom one regards as one's equal with one's views while awaiting a response that might involve disagreement and the need to reconsider one's position. The move generated the possibility of viewing knowledge as an ongoing project rather than as a given text or a revelation. It therefore heralded humans' gradually improving ability to understand and control their environment. But the open conversation's benefits, Popper concedes, were not unambiguous. As a third-world phenomenon, science is not controlled by anyone and accordingly confronts us with an unpredictable future: nobody is ever in charge and everyone is affected. By contrast, closed-society ontology was reassuring to its holders. It allowed them to live in an immutable world that demands no further reflection. Every person organically belonged to a collective whole, leaving no gap between subjectivity and objectivity, no nagging doubt about one's worth or life-ends and no existential angst (Popper, 1966 v. 1: 57–59).

Why did anyone exchange such stability for the constant unease of a debate that installs uncertainty, undermines one's most cherished values and encourages the expression of troubling differences? Popper names travel and the ensuing exposure to different worldviews as a trigger, first to curiosity, then to doubt, and consequently to dialogue (Popper, 1966 v. 1: 60). But the sequence could have taken an opposing direction. The relativity of worldviews engendered by travel could have made individuals and communities more defensive and hostile when facing perceived threats to their beliefs. Why is it feasible to assume that the availability of discussion was enough for it to be chosen over isolation, war and repression?

Winnicott may address this gap. The requirement of an object to relate to precedes and infuses other motivations. But for relations with that object to be healthy and rewarding, the object has to be another subject, a fully human other who is like the self but consists beyond the self's control. Transitional space and the play activities based on it express the recognition of the other person's autonomy. Rolling the ball over to the parent, the child's agency anticipates confirmation by another individual: the ball is rolled back by a person rather than bouncing from a wall. The velocity or angle of the incoming throw cannot be predicted by the player, as it emanates from another human. Validation of the self by another person, the primary good sought by all, is achieved by allowing for the uncontrollable agency of others. Play grants us the synergy of autonomy and recognition (Winnicott, 1991: 99).

Such a form of validation is unlikely to be found in the closed society, where received beliefs are expressed through repetitive rituals and habitual compliance (Popper, 1966 v. 1: 172–173). Its residents cannot convey their thoughts to anyone who does not already share them. Like the very young child to whom the parent seems unconditionally available, members of the closed society may be assured of being continuous with their surroundings, but they gain no recognition as autonomous authors of cognition and action. By contrast, the reciprocal examination of myths that founds the open society provides that good and therefore responds to a constitutive human need. In that first open conversation, each participant tossed their own tale, which was, in turn, tossed back as questions were directed at it. Then, the participants traded places, with a new storyteller offering their myth to be questioned. Tolerance and the expression of difference were not experienced only as a frightful loss of equilibrium. They were, instead, pleasurable, as they granted each person their first opportunity of receiving recognition in the form of comment, criticism and correction.

The second motivational question arising from Popper's account has to do with maintaining the open society once established. Popper expects a new ethics to form once myth is abandoned and the open society arises. Our acts no longer follow from a given cosmos. We cannot be told in advance what is wrong and right for us to do, and we cannot be exonerated from moral agonizing by following given guidelines and performing known rites. Without the overarching scheme of a comprehensive knowledge system to fall back on, we have to judge for ourselves, which encourages a reflective and considerate posture. As each person is burdened with the weight of their own actions, the open society forgoes the single-minded intolerance of the closed one. It becomes infused with an ethics that restrains individual conduct without undue recourse to coercion and sanctions: 'it is we, and we alone, who are responsible' (Popper, 1966 v. 1: 66). But it is not clear how this assumption of individual responsibility takes hold and how it can survive for long. Where no comprehensive philosophy tells people what is wrong and right, why should a sense of personal responsibility become prevalent? Would individuals not rather assert themselves while suffering no compunction except for weakness and failure?

Again, Winnicott may offer the outline for an answer. The empowering realization that others are subjects like us and can validate our contribution entails acknowledging that they are vulnerable like us. With awareness of the mother's independent personhood arrives the insight that the recipient of the child's love is the same person as the recipient of the child's aggression. Following the course of healthy integration, Winnicott (1984: 206) expects, the self becomes able 'to appreciate the personality of the mother figure, and this has the tremendously important result that he is concerned as to the results of his instinctual experience, physical and ideational'. These results have to do with perceived harm to the mother: while resilient, she is capable of suffering. Both resilience and suffering emanate from her being a person with a continuity in time and space. The child's guilt comes from a similar appreciation of the self's continuity and hence responsibility for the past. The ability to feel guilt is born. Healthy individuality is inseparable from regret over the harm inevitably done within the relationship, and from the wish to repair it. Concern for other people appears simultaneously with the capacity for creative agency (Winnicott, 1984: 91–96, 262–277, 1986: 80–89). Free individuals assume responsibility to others as part and parcel of their freedom. The open society can be assured of its moral and public cohesion as its free and equal members are endowed with a commitment to others acquired alongside their sense of agency.

The complementary relationship between Popper and Winnicott cuts both ways. If Winnicott points to the sources of the individual motivation entailed by Popper's account of the open society, then Popper's grounding of third-world systems in evolution lends credibility to Winnicott's belief in the rise of play as a historical novelty. Winnicott ascribes a contextual character to his developmental model. That model can only function, he suspects, in a specific historical phase. Prior to it, most civilizations perceived the cosmos as given and demanded performance of fixed roles that accorded with that perception. There was no concept of a distinct personal interior that could present its surroundings with anything new. While games technically existed, substantial play did not. All forms of communication were rigidly structured. 'We cannot', Winnicott comments, 'easily identify…with the men and women of early times who… identified themselves with the community and with nature' (Winnicott, 1991: 70). Winnicott speculates that science may have introduced the distinction between subject and object, and so awakened humans to the possibility of examining and using their environment rather than complying with what they thought were its demands. The dawning realization that they were thinking subjects with their own internal lives enabled humans to conceive of questioning and impacting their surroundings, generating the personal creativity that psychoanalytic theory would come to equate with health (Winnicott, 1991: 70). But such a reading simply defers the question: science could not be the source of the subject-object distinction as science's own work requires a foundation in the ability to challenge and investigate. How could such abilities materialize in the archaic communities Winnicott thinks preceded modernity?

A clue may be found if the resolution level is broadened from psychology to sociology and its interface with biology, as Popper suggests. The potential for creating third-world phenomena is independent of specific historical circumstances. Language, a system controlled by none but affected by all, appears in all civilizations. As they grant humans the ability to consider solutions for survival problems before actually trying them and possibly perishing in the process, language, writing, scholarly reflection and scientific research can all be regarded as evolutionary devices: 'the third world is a natural product of the human animal, comparable to a spider's web' (Popper, 1979: 112). For this particular species, then, the potential is in principle available at any point for an open-ended dialogue between participants who adhere to the rules of the exchange as if these rules were a given reality. Open societies actively pursue this exchange, but the venue for it exists in a dormant state in the closed society as well.

The rigidity of the closed society, where innovation is hindered, is an artificial imposition over a universal, nature-based trait rather than a default option. Received certainty is a crust that can be fractured by the first hint of doubt or discrepancy. Once a frank conversation commences, the third-world dynamic asserts itself. The conversation generates new knowledge that is hard to repress, as it is independent from any particular exponent. 'Innocence once lost', Popper remarks, 'cannot be regained' (1966 v. 1: 182). Dialogue, which for Winnicott would be play and play-like activities, among mutually recognizing individual subjects may emerge within the archaic, closed society, despite that society's worst intentions. Winnicott's assumption of a historical break that allowed the psychoanalytical model of the mind to form thus gains a likelihood not fully accounted for by Winnicott's own work. Added to the parallels between Popper's and Winnicott's ideas, their reciprocal complementarity further suggests that they share a rationale whose outline exceeds its manifestations in their separate works.

Privacy and Civic Engagement in the Open Society

Popper and Winnicott place individual agency centre-stage and task society's political arms with assuring the conditions for it to form and thrive. The third-world conversation of scholars and scientists and the transitional space that opens up between child and parent are alike sites where individual liberty unfolds. They therefore merit the respect and protection of societal institutions, as both authors claim. The ensuing political model seems to match with the conventionally liberal view of democracy, in which social institutions are organized around the core value of individual freedom. However, Popper and Winnicott differ at some points from the liberal variants grounded in the thought of early modernity and the nineteenth century.

Individualist liberals like Locke and J.S. Mill concurred on the necessity of distinguishing between the area where people can follow their own discretion, and the region marked for the collective action performed by governmental bodies. Individuals should be free to make a certain range of choices. The activities and sites ordered by these choices – families, businesses, voluntary associations, and the expression of opinion in literature and the press – should be immune to governmental intervention. At the same time, government, as the policing agent tasked with the private sphere's safety, should be structured by impersonal principles so as to preserve itself from the partial desires of the private realm (Fawcett, 2014; Ryan, 2012).

Alongside these dominant, individualist variants of liberalism, a pluralist approach developed that proposed a different way of protecting privacy and politics from each other. Authors like Edmund Burke, Lord Acton and J.N. Figgis were troubled by the possibility that the constitutional and representative bodies entrusted by individualist liberalism might damage the texture of the multiple, familiar, everyday environments that provide people with the experience of stability and personal significance. As they were made deliberately anonymous by individualist liberalism's commitment to impartiality, bureaucracy and legislation could not respect the street-level particularities necessary for the life of groups and associations. Accordingly, this pluralist strand suggests that voluntary private associations should be given standing against government: individual rights are to be supplemented by group rights, so as to interpose a legally recognized layer of social sites between individual and state. But if pluralists configured the sphere division differently from individualists, they retained it nonetheless. Whether neatly partitioned from government's reach by individual entitlement or buffered away from the state by intermediary bodies, privacy keeps its shielded quality in both liberal schools, while civic participation and politics keep their impersonal and juristic character (Levy, 2015).

Popper and Winnicott appear to reconcile the individualist emphasis on freedom as an ability to express opinions and wishes, and the pluralist trust in the ability of intermediary, voluntary and communal sites to grant their participants a sense of direction and stability. But the perception of freedom Popper and Winnicott share does not stay within the fixed bounds of a designated private realm. For both authors, liberty is not fulfilled by the capability to act on individual discretion. It takes place in a setting that changes its participants, and consequently impacts the civic sphere as well. In Popper and Winnicott alike, the trajectory is enabled by two features they ascribe to the third world and to transitional space: their self-regulating peacefulness, and their generative, productive capacity.

For Popper (1979: 146–148), the open society's founding discussion is driven by the quest for knowledge, itself an offshoot of an evolutionary process that propels all animals to seek solutions to survival problems. Each separate discipline and subfield that ensue develops its own rules, but all are committed to the universal search for truth. If we engage in a discussion in order to get nearer to the truth and so enhance our understanding of the world we live in, then we also believe that the truth exists and that we can decipher at least some of its aspects by comparing notes and correcting them in accordance with that comparison: the discussion moves towards coherence. While suspending final judgement, the participants adhere to 'the unscientific, the metaphysical faith in laws, in regularities which we can uncover' (Popper, 1972: 278). When claims cannot reconcile by reference to such laws, the discussants await further inputs instead of forcing closure, as such closure would harm coherence (Popper, 1966 v. 2: 224–226, 1972: 280). The conversation, then, is preceded by its participants' commitment to a shared end, to that end's coherence and to the avoidance of imposition. The encounter of equal subjectivities in open debate regulates itself and avoids resort to coercion.

Popper anticipates the rejoinder that the orderly debate of scholars does not exhaust our freely chosen activities. Not all private action can rely on internal regulation. The high stakes involved in raising a family, maintaining a business or pursuing a career press upon their participants what they sense are objective threats to lifeline, property or progeny. This often precludes tolerance. Empowering force-wielding institutions to mediate between the individuals who confront each other in the private sphere, Popper (2002: 471) concedes, remains a regrettable necessity. A civic, political realm where final decisions over punishing crimes and fighting enemies are made is therefore part of Popper's scheme. Its rationale includes arbitrary closure and the use of force, and therefore contrasts with the peaceful self-regulation of open conversation. But the status of the enforcing institutions in the open society is contingent rather than essential. Third-world phenomena are not static. They constantly develop. Each debate unleashes further debates, with new disciplines covering more areas. As third-world phenomena expand, they amplify the evolutionary trend towards substituting reflection for pain and risk. With physical survival becoming less precarious, individuals are less likely to commit desperate acts for ensuring it. The coercive aspect of the public realm recedes. Social life is no longer underlined by fear and is thereby less prone to the divisions fear causes, along with the dogmatic ideologies that cater to these divisions. Civic engagement takes on the quality of consensually managing concrete problems (Popper, 2008: 360–369). A transfer occurs in the open society 'from the realm of ideology to that of social engineering' (Popper, 2008: 392).

With coercion and violence ebbing, political bodies become accessible to the influence of science and philosophy, whose development accelerates under political freedom. Popper (2002: 474–475) expects the habits and practices of scholarly exchange to incrementally replace the moody vagaries of public opinion and diminish the significance of the assemblies that register public opinion's preferences, controversies and struggles. When open-society conversations proceed freely, a rough agreement forms around the realization, brought about by the experience of engaging in them, that humans can regulate themselves to a degree that makes violence redundant and peace a universal aspiration (Popper, 2008: 303). The bodies entrusted with policing and security decline in significance through the operation of an expanding private sphere. Rather than distinguishing itself from the various intersubjective encounters at the core of that sphere, the open society's civic arena acquires these discussions' qualities. The difference between the spheres blurs. A liberal civilization crystallizes in which open-ended, creative and self-regulating exchanges occur at all levels.

Playing and Citizenship

A comparable perception of the intersubjective meeting as self-regulating and expanding is entailed in Winnicott's theory. Like Popper, Winnicott does not envisage a world without politics, states, governments and borders. The inevitable failures of early holding see to that, as when they are translated into the big numbers of entire societies they engender disorder and violence, and so call for institutions to tackle them (Winnicott, 1986: 34, 212–219, 233, 243–246, 257–258). But, like Popper, Winnicott expects the peacefully self-regulating and creative features of the intersubjective arena to mitigate the harshness of public life.

Play fosters communication and motor skills, contributing to a sense of agency that reconciles the child to the concept of external reality. In a similar way, play renders the encounter with social rules a rewarding one. If the parent were to throw the ball out of the window rather than toss it back, the child's agency would be denied and the game's rationale undermined. If the child were to do the same, the parent would revert to a mere projection of the child's imagination. By contrast, Winnicott (1991: 41) emphasizes that play is not fantasy or magic: it consists of doing, rather than imagining, because it takes constraints and liabilities into account. Maintaining the rules of the game bolsters agency and relatedness. The acceptance of structure cultivates one's autonomy rather than impinges on it (Winnicott, 1986: 40–49). Accordingly, encounters and activities that take place in transitional space abide by internal rules without recourse to external policing. Since social interaction is not experienced as the imposition of confining laws over personal desire, the aggression arising from seeing others as threats need not be prevalent.

For Winnicott, play is a form of behaviour learned during very early childhood. It is, at the same time, a natural activity grounded in physiological characters and biological facts (Winnicott, 1988: 26–29). Health consists in an integrated functioning of the abilities based on these characters. The ability to achieve it can be encouraged or harmed by the conditions generated by social institutions, but its potentiality is independent of these institutions. Health and play are therefore part of humanity's natural state. As it is self-regulating, play includes the ability to contain, resolve and utilize conflict. As it is natural, it is authentic and receives a normative priority over societal institutions. Winnicott thus avoids the danger inherent to state-of-nature ideologies of valorizing an unmediated, raw and potentially unsettling 'authenticity': when actualized through transitional activities nature is already civilized (Bowker, 2017).

Transitional activities are, moreover, expansive. Play is the template for all healthy converse with society. Progressing from parents to siblings, neighbours, peer groups and colleagues, play becomes art, sports, literature, philosophy, science, commercial venture and community work. In each arena, individuals stake out meanings that are significant to them so that these meanings can be reacted upon by others, thus offering validation to the self (Winnicott, 1986: 35–36, 1991: 95–103). The space where individual agency is experienced and becomes real to us, then, resides in the multiple everyday arenas where people gain and give recognition (Winnicott, 1986: 247). These include families; workplaces; villages; towns; churches; professional bodies; and voluntary associations, such as 'perhaps the local bowls club' (Winnicott, 1991: 141).

The experiences of interacting with concrete others within multiple, overlapping and rule-structured sites inform a public whose attention, when called to bear on formal politics, attaches to concrete candidates rather than to idolized leader figures. These candidates are other human subjects who can be related to as such. Public attention similarly attaches to concrete issues one can try to resolve through engagement with others rather than to pre-packaged, rigid ideologies (Winnicott, 1986: 249–250). As one converses with imperfect other humans, from the vulnerable parent onwards, friction is accepted and tolerated as accompanying all relationships. Intimate harmony is not contrasted with the irreconcilable clash that supposedly occurs among strangers. All organizational levels are extensions of the family (Winnicott, 1986: 27).

This position differentiates Winnicott from Fairbairn. For both, the ability to recognize others, and thus be recognized, involves accepting one's indebtedness. Fairbairn's account follows on Hegel, for whom the burden of reparation becomes heavier with expanding social bonds. In the ultimate, final bond – that of citizen and state – that debt can entail sacrificing one's life as a necessary price for actualizing humans' capacities that the state embodies. Fairbairn accordingly emphasizes the ability to shoulder the impersonal and often dangerous duties of citizen and soldier as expressions of the healthy, tolerably integrated personality who transcends the infantilizing pull of the internal objects. For Winnicott, too, the recognition of the other requires relinquishing omnipotence and is expressed by conceding one's dependence on others. Saying 'thank you', Winnicott (1984: 230) writes, points to the child's acknowledgement of indebtedness.

But by offering his account of transitional activity, Winnicott adds a plane of relationships where recognition of one's limits and concession of other's independent existence are sensed as validating to the self. The circle of contacts, interactions and venues for acting on one's agency widens through play-based activities that may differ in the level of emotional intensity they call upon, but do not exert the abnegation that Hegel's scheme implies. The reward, rather than just the debt incurred, grows with these activities' expansion. There is no necessary horizon of ultimate sacrifice, as in Hegel. With every additional site of interaction, individuals gather more skills, more connections, more potentiality for developing and implementing internally generated contents. Play and play-based activities aggregate into culture and form a shared pool of practices and ideas to which all may contribute and from which all may draw. That culture then benefits from the inputs of its creative individual constituents. The contents are made meaningful by the terms of that culture, like a move within a game is meaningful by the game's rules. Such contributions lead to further growth. The entire process is rooted in the ability to play gained in early childhood:

> [I]n any cultural field, *it is not possible to be original except on a basis of tradition*. Conversely, no one in the line of cultural contributors repeats except as a deliberate quotation, and the unforgiveable sin in the cultural field is plagiarism. The interplay between originality and the acceptance of tradition as the basis for inventiveness seems to me to be just one more example...of the interplay between separateness and union.
>
> (Winnicott, 1991: 99)

The healthy, creative self-fulfilment that both asserts autonomy and acknowledges dependence is available through this cultural experience rather than through the obligations of citizenship and state. If the politics of states, armies, police forces and governments remains indispensable because of the holding environment's fragility, that kind of politics and the institutions where it plays out are not essential for human fulfilment, as they express no special, indispensable psychic capacity. In its final horizon, culture is a world phenomenon that transcends borders and lends humans their sense of belonging to a shared, layered solidarity that combines common traditions and the possibility of innovation and advance (Winnicott, 1986: 60).

Winnicott's work thus echoes the potentiality named by Popper for the gradual, if never complete, displacement of civic publicity by habits and practices that extend and replicate the simultaneously protected and transformative interactions of the private sphere. That potentiality is germane to both authors' perception of freedom as acquired through an encounter that generates its own rules. By organizing their understandings of democracy around this perception of personal freedom, Popper and Winnicott differ from both the individualist and the pluralist renditions of liberalism. For these earlier, more established forms of liberal and democratic thought, the fulfilment gained in the private sphere had to be separated from the civic sphere either by legal individual rights or by the addition of an intermediary layer of groups and associations that contrasts with the impartiality of law and government. In both variants, politics remained a specialized, unique activity that had to be strictly distinguished from the emotion and particularity of the private realm. For Popper and Winnicott, by contrast, the liberty assured in the private sphere develops to circumvent, influence and in some ways diminish the realm of formal politics.

Conclusion

While moored to differing disciplines and methods, Popper's and Winnicott's concepts share some significant features. Popper's third world and Winnicott's transitional space denote sites where interactions take place that hand their participants the ability to move beyond the closed circle of their received beliefs and subjective minds, and negotiate with the demands of objective reality. In both cases, reasonable leverage over reality and a corresponding experience of agency for the self are gained by encountering another self who is recognized and respected as such. These encounters instil a rule-abiding, morally concerned and peaceful attitude. The combination of lawful peacefulness and creative freedom entails that activities based on these sites multiply and expand, and that their self-structuring character expands with them. The political world may itself be influenced by this process, and consequently shed off some of its association with coercion and violence. Both authors envision public bodies that enhance and imitate, rather than merely complement, the transformative interaction that occurs through sociable, collegiate and cultural activities.

Consequently, if Popper and Winnicott maintain liberalism's emphasis on individual freedom as a desired end around which the societal order should organize itself, their perception of liberty differs from earlier, individualist and pluralist variants of liberalism. The earlier liberal strands distinguished the private world where personal liberty is enjoyed from the civic and political sphere where collective decisions on the use of force are taken. Popper and Winnicott, by contrast, view the intersubjective encounters that occupy the position of a shielded private sphere in their accounts as harbouring the potentiality of changing the urgency level and the contents of politics. As the exchanges of the third world and transitional space allow their participants to acknowledge and utilize their differences, a narrower potentiality for actual destruction remains, toning down the levels of violence in the entire society.

If Popper struck a chord with his midcentury audience by reframing democracy as the open society, and if Winnicott similarly resonated with his readership by casting Klein's gloomy account as harbouring the prospects for creativity and growth, then this resonance may have to do with their ability to touch a broader contemporary agreement. Their shared features align with the vision of a free, diverse and peaceful society advanced by welfare-oriented liberals as well as by some of their detractors on right and left. The recurrence of these themes in several disciplinary and ideological frameworks hints at an emerging consensus that expected the developing private sphere, whatever the specific contents attributed to it, to impact, educate and shape, if not obviate, the practices involved in the politics of national governments, formal citizenship and power struggle. Through Winnicott's contribution, therefore, object relations theory can be understood as a constituent of a midcentury sensibility that acquired democracy and liberalism with new meanings.

References

Alexander, S. (2012). Primary maternal preoccupation: D.W. Winnicott and social democracy in mid-twentieth-century Britain. In Alexander, S., and Taylor, B. (eds.), *History and psyche: Culture, psychoanalysis, and the past.* New York: Palgrave, 149–172.

Beveridge, W.H. (1940). *Peace by federation?* London: Federal Union.

Beveridge, W.H. (1945). *The price of peace.* London: Pilot.

Bowker, M.H. (2017). Safety in danger and privation: Ambivalent fantasies of natural states invoked in reaction to loss. In Bowker, M.H., and Buzby, A. (eds.), *D.W. Winnicott and political theory.* New York: Palgrave, 137–162.

Carr, E.H. (1945). *Nationalism and after.* London: Macmillan.

Fairbairn, W.R.D. (1952). *Psycho-analytic studies of the personality.* London: Tavistock.

Fawcett, E. (2014). *Liberalism: The life of an idea.* Princeton, NJ: Princeton University Press.

Guntrip, H. (2001). *Schizoid phenomena, object-relations and the self.* London: Karnac.

Hacohen, M.H. (2000). *Karl Popper – The formative years, 1920–1945.* Cambridge: Cambridge University Press.

Hayek, F.A. (2007). *The road to serfdom.* Chicago, IL: Chicago University Press.

Hayek, F.A. (2011.) *The constitution of liberty.* Chicago, IL: University of Chicago Press.

Hoggett, P. (2008). Relational thinking and welfare practice. In Clarke, S., Hahn, H., and Hoggett, P. (eds.), *Object relations and social relations.* London: Karnac, 65–86.

Holthaus, L. (2014). G.D.H. Cole's international thought: The dilemmas of justifying socialism in the twentieth century. *The International History Review* 36 (5): 858–875.

Laing, R.D. (1965). *The divided self.* Harmondsworth: Penguin.

Lamb, P. (2004). *Harold Laski.* New York: Palgrave Macmillan.

Laski, H.J. (1938). *A grammar of politics*, Fourth Edition. London: Allen and Unwin.

Laski, H.J. (1943). *Reflections on the revolution of our time.* New York: Viking.

Levy, J.T. (2015). *Rationalism, pluralism, andfreedom.* Oxford: Oxford University Press.

Mitrany, D. (1943). *A working peace system.* London: The Royal Institute of International Affairs.

Nachman, D.L. (1981). Psychoanalysis and social theory: The origin of society and of guilt. *Salmagundi* 52/53: 65–106.

Popper, K.R. (1966). *The open society and its enemies.* Princeton, NJ: Princeton University Press.

Popper, K.R. (1972). *The logic of scientific discovery*, 6th impression. London: Hutchinson.

Popper, K.R (1979). *Objective knowledge*, revised edition. Oxford: Clarendon.

Popper, K.R. (2002). *Conjectures and refutations.* New York and London: Routledge.

Press.Popper, K.R. (2008). *After the open society.* London and New York: Routledge.

Rieff, P. (1966). *The triumph of the therapeutic.* New York: Harper and Row.

Rosenboim, O. (2017). *The emergence of globalism.* Princeton, NJ: Princeton University Press.

Rustin, M. (1991). *The good society and the inner world.* London and New York: Verso.

Ryan, A. (2012). *The making of modern liberalism.* Princeton, NJ: Princeton University Press.

Shearmur, J. (1996). *The political thought of Karl Popper.* London and New York: Routledge.

Stokes, G. (1998). *Popper.* Cambridge: Polity.

Wallace, E.R. (1992). Freud and the mind-body problem. In Gelfand, T., and Kerr, J. (eds.), *Freud and the history of psychoanalysis.* Hillsdale, NJ: The Analytic Press, 231–269.

Winnicott, D.W. (1965). *The maturational processes and the facilitating environment.* London: Hogarth.

Winnicott, D.W. (1984). *Through paediatrics to psychoanalysis.* London: Karnac.
Winnicott, D.W. (1986). *Home is where we start from.* New York and London: W.W. Norton.
Winnicott, D.W. (1988). *Human nature.* Philadelphia, PA: Brunner/Mazel.
Winnicott, D.W. (1991). *Playing and reality.* London: Routledge.

6 Jessica Benjamin and the Consequences of Maternal Agency

If Winnicott's affinity with Popper illustrates the British analysts' concurrence with their time's rising, if implicit, new expectations from the politics of democracy, then Jessica Benjamin's work can concretize the British school's long-term legacy as a political theory. The ideological dimension involved in the works of most midcentury object relations authors is usually implicit. The Sutties, Fairbairn and Winnicott were not primarily political thinkers: while having specific ideas about public life, their main focus remained psychological and therapy-related. But an expressly political and ideological theory based on object relations insights has been provided by Jessica Benjamin since the 1980s. It combines a feminist reading of object relations theory along with Hegelian philosophy and other inputs into a comprehensive social outlook. In Benjamin's work, accordingly, the ideological legacy of object relations theory, along with its potentialities and vulnerabilities, stands out in sharper relief than in most other contributions.

Benjamin argues that the capacity to act as a self-directing and healthily confident individual proceeds from the child's recognition of the mother as another human subject who both cares for the child and exercises her own independent agency. Robust individuality includes acknowledging the existence of another, autonomous yet vulnerable subject. The conditions of parental holding, then, become crucial for a polity based on the assumption of self-directing, free citizens. The mother's well-being and sense of personal agency are central for that polity. Conversely, the child's development into creative and communicative individuality cannot fully take place if the mother is experienced as a passive, immobile object of another's desire. In a patriarchal civilization that relegates women to inferiority, the full potentiality of healthy growth cannot be realized. The patriarchal family setting instils children with a concept of power hierarchy before it allows them to form a sense of individual agency. Any subsequent notion of personal identity is processed in terms of having power over someone else rather than in the terms of relating to someone else. Patriarchy, along with its perceptions of personal freedom, is pervaded by inequality, domination and conflict, which are broadly accepted under these conditions as the default option of human life.

Social philosophies that analyze society in terms of irresoluble differences that require force and conflict normalize the pathologies of this civilization by presenting them as just the politics that can be had.

Benjamin's work is extensively debated among psychologists, feminist critics, political scientists, cultural theorists and other commentators. Benjamin (1998: 82–84, 2000) has occasionally joined that debate to refine some of her messages and correct misreadings. She has been commended for weaving a rich theory of democratic deliberation, akin to that of Hannah Arendt, that takes into account the preverbal aspects of social relations (Meehan, 2002). This allows Benjamin to escape the overly rationalist assumptions of theorists such as Jürgen Habermas, for whom social dialogue occurs exclusively in the consciously verbal plane of communication. From Benjamin's perspective, the early, preverbal ingredients of our personalities do not detract from the value of deliberation but lend it a constitutive value, as they allow politics to express, enrich and transform broader aspects of our personalities than can be expressed through formally verbal communication. Benjamin's work has at the same time incurred criticism, as her turn to what looks like the primordially emotional groundwork of interpersonal exchange appears to justify a retreat from reason and thereby undermine any recognizably rational social order. Christopher Lasch (1984) numbers Benjamin among the id-authors, who, as he sees it, advocate a Dionysian, protean perception of human liberty that abandons responsibility and complexity. Such approaches, Lasch thinks, eliminate the distinction between desire, conscience and social discipline. These distinctions, Lasch (240–244, 258–259) holds, form the one attribute that rescues humans from being either animals or slaves.

As an alternative to such interpretations, I suggest that Benjamin's political theory fleshes out the potentialities embedded in the observations of the earlier object relations authors. These allow for complexity and tension: at their best, relationships and subjectivities are 'messy' (Benjamin, 1999: 199). As in Winnicott, some structuring is required as the basis of substantial freedom. As, moreover, occurs in other object relations-based political thought, Benjamin's attribution of self-regulating, benevolent and creativity-inducing potentialities to the dynamics of a healthy early-family setting results in a diminishment of the formally egalitarian institutions that constitutional democracies rely on. Consequently, Benjamin's political theory is neither as anarchic as her critics suggests nor as compatible with constitutional democratic institutions as her more supportive readers claim: it is instead one in which the civic sphere gradually gives way to a complex but benevolent private sphere.

In what follows I first describe the setting in which the American relational school, to which Benjamin belongs, has taken form. I then focus on Benjamin's theory of maturation and gender, arguing that it bridges several lacunas in the philosophical thought with which it converses.

Next, I note the difficulties involved in Benjamin's worldview, paying attention mainly to the interlinked persistence within it of gender, on the one hand, and to the diminishment of the civic realm, on the other hand.

The Relational School: From Objectivity to Dialogue

The American relational group that includes authors like Lewis Aron, Nancy Chodorow, Jay Greenberg and Stephen Mitchell, among others, emerged in the 1970s and established itself consequently as a distinct school with its own methods and affiliations. While drawing ideas from earlier American theorists like Harry Sullivan and international authors like Erich Fromm, the relational school sees the British object relations approach as a main inspiration. The infant's need for relating, as emphasized in object relations literature, impacts lifelong patterns, as perceived responses to that need are imbibed and consequently structure the individual's internal landscape. Therapists are required not only to enable their patients to understand these patterns, but also to experience a hopeful relationship as a corrective to the psychic vulnerabilities acquired earlier in life. Integration of various emotional states into a functioning and relating personality serves within the relational school as the standard of healthy development (Mitchell and Aron, 1999).

The relational school grappled with a different context than the one in which Ian Suttie, Jane Suttie, Fairbairn and Winnicott had worked. Removed from the midcentury's experiences of battling industrial poverty and totalitarian armies, the intellectual and public debate of the 1960s shifted to the angst of the Cold War, the inequalities and frustrations of an increasingly global capitalist order, and the discontents of a competitive and alienated society. Psychoanalysis, additionally, encountered its own challenges. No longer the novelty it had been in the early twentieth century, Freudian nomenclature was now somewhat of an ossified tradition. In terms of content, psychoanalysis was criticized for equating health with conformity to social expectations and for clinging to outdated assumptions about the family and sexual roles. In terms of validity and therapeutic application, analysis was overshadowed by advances in neuroscience and the broader fields of medical research (Hale, 1995). A largely private practice in the United States, psychoanalysis also faced competition from alternative counselling methods like behavioural therapy and coaching.

The relational school reflects these concerns. Deploying insights from the British theorists, it focuses on the mother's role and the child's quest for relating, holding and validation, thus distancing itself from the rigid and hierarchic resonance of Freud's model while allowing more flexibility in treatment than the taxonomies of ego psychology could enable. Responding to its milieu and its paying clients, the late twentieth-century relational approach stresses the role of the therapist as a human who recognizes the particular patient's inputs and shuns simplifying them to fit an abstract model. Consequently, relational analysis can provide an attentive psychodynamic treatment that avoids orthodox therapy's stiff detachment, behavioural treatment's sense of mechanic conditioning and object relations theory's alleged tendency of perceiving adults as children. Relational clinicians meet their clients as equals who can openly challenge the therapist's own position in the relationship. The focus on conversation and subjective meaning absolves the American school from the pretension to being a positivist discipline that might compare unfavourably to medical and other empirical and quantitatively validated research (Berman, 1997).

The relational school openly discusses its ideological motivations and their anchoring in a specific historical setting. In the decades following the Second World War, the form of constitutional and democratic governance embodied by the United States could boast its global dominance and economic prosperity, and present itself as a beacon of both sincere morality and material success. But social critics were already warning that American democracy failed to deliver in significant ways. Even when ignoring the many places where it strayed from its declared principles, the American polity was organized for protecting a mainly negative perception of liberty, aligning with free-market legislation and a capitalist work ethic. Its aridly individualist notion of equality allowed intercommunal inequalities to fester, with minorities and cultural enclaves constantly marginalized. A supposedly impartial legalism teamed up with the similarly impartial calculations of profit to set up a grid in which differences in personal sensibility, viewpoint, gender, culture or economic clout did not openly register and could not be discussed, admitted or criticized. Individuals were granted a narrowly defined equal freedom at the price of conforming to corporate discipline, denying their inner desires and turning their backs on communal and social loyalties. Parts of each subjectivity were neglected in the same way that some constituents of the society were. Classical analysis and its American, ego-psychology variants colluded with the surrounding culture by stressing the universal structures of personality and the matching, objective and emotionally distant, authority of the analyst (Seligman, 2019).

Under these conditions, object relations theory's premises allowed progressive-minded psychologists to pivot away from Freud's positivism. Object relations theory posits attachment, recognition and love rather than physical satisfaction as the basic goods. As these goods are not material, they do not create scarcity and therefore liberate psychology from the scarcity-based, hydraulic model in which a fixed space may contain a fixed quantity of pressure. As Flax (1990: 55–56) notes, object relations theory evaded the reduction of minds to the mechanic rationale of capitalism. Moreover, with object relations theory's emphasis on the mind as responding to an internalized model of society, the self could be conceived of as normally and even healthily multiple, heterogeneous and diverse, as illustrated by Winnicott's notion of cross-identification. The advance beyond the monadic positivism of ego psychology aligned with emerging cultural and political sensibilities (Flax, 1981).

At the same time, however, object relations theory invited modification. Object relations theory upheld integration as an ideal, finding a place for destruction and aggression as well as for love in the child's journey towards healthy adulthood. This notion of integration concurred with the cultural climate of the midcentury, where the polity committed itself to providing all its citizens and all its classes with the means for a dignified existence from the cradle to the grave. While allowing internal plurality, this notion of integration seemed to suggest a comprehensive, systemic finality as its ultimate reference point. The welfare state could build public accommodation because it had a clear notion of how a standard household looked like, knowing in advance how many rooms families need, how their members spend their time together, how they interface with their neighbours. Bowlby, Fairbairn and Winnicott could advise state institutions, families and individuals alike, because they had a clear view of how the home mutually accommodates to its members, and what its relationship to the surrounding society should be. In the second half of the century, by contrast, it became increasingly difficult to retain such certainties. Cultural and social forms proliferated and could no longer be addressed by a standard package of services. Different communities had different ideas of well-being. Varying templates of sexuality, conjugal bonding and household organization gained legitimacy and were becoming publicly visible. Educated sensibilities favoured this multiplicity as a form of liberal egalitarianism, as it offered equal consideration to every social constituent. Multiplicity rather than the reciprocal completion of different constituents was now the ideal.

Correspondingly, the notions of valid knowledge and science were changing. In the midcentury setting in which object relations theory was formulated, economists, sociologists, accountants, doctors and psychologists could participate in social planning because their disciplines provided solid standards that cohered into a unified system. But that perception of knowledge was increasingly placed in doubt. The more pluralist attitude to knowledge that ensued informed the formation of the American relational school. Stephen Mitchell was instrumental in highlighting the continuity between object relations thought and the American relational group. However, when describing the trends that informed the rise of the American approach, Mitchell (2003: 68–76) describes a general drift towards relativity and the blurring of lines between object and subject, mind and matter, specialist and client. Among other developments, the discovery of neuroplasticity suggested that the mind impacts its materially biological basis in the body as well as the other way around, as neuronic paths reroute according to inputs from thinking consciousness. Such developments meshed in with the ideological concern for acknowledging the equality of groups and cultures as well as of individuals: the multiplicity of groups hinted at the relativity of valid knowledge, including therapeutic knowledge. That knowledge was posited in the analyst, resulting from study, training and experience, but it also came from the patient, whose cognitions and emotions could no longer be assumed to be wholly external to the analyst's thought and sensations: object was impacting subject as much as the reverse (Westerman, 2005).

Processing these concerns, relational analysts focuses on an ambivalence that arises from the object relations view. Object relations authors like Ian Suttie, Winnicott and Guntrip had echoed Ferenczi's notion of healing love. If the patient is constantly motivated to maintain a relationship with an internalized mother figure, then the analyst can, in orthodox fashion, help the patient explore the instances where that effort disrupts adult life. But as the patient needs relating rather than just knowledge, then the analyst should also provide the patient with an instance of a nourishing and trustworthy relationship. Analytic expertise heals, but it heals through relating. While conceding this point, object relations theory persisted in its insistence on the structured character of treatment. The analyst's stable posture has to be trusted if therapy is to be a holding space where the patient can go through the work required for therapy. The patient can fruitfully regress, for example, only in the space held by the analyst, as the stability of that space is itself therapeutic. And once set in motion, the processes that the patient goes through are analyzed as arising solely from that patient's personality and psychic past. The analyst, Winnicott (1984: 286) stresses, is an enabler, not a contributor, and should abide by the strict rules entailed by this mandate: 'the whole thing adds up to the fact that the analyst *behaves* himself or herself'.

However, if the analyst performs as a particular other person who treats the patient through the very fact of relating, then analytic work has to include the analyst's inputs as such, and these inputs show in the contents offered by the patient. These contents, then, should be viewed as more than an elaboration on an internal world carried around by the patient alone. When analyzing, the therapist has to analyze his or her own position as a subject. The theorists of the American relational school focus on this point. As relating is valued for its source in another person, the flawed humanity of the analyst should be treated as a therapeutic resource as much as that analyst's skill. The therapist's emotional, motoric and verbal responses to the patient become analytically significant, as do the therapist's frailty, absences and occasional failure. The focus expands from attention to the patient's past to the present of the clinic where patient and clinician mutually attune, even if this includes what for Winnicott would be analytic misbehaviour. Their attunement exceeds the technicality of transference and counter transference, as the patient calibrates towards the particular therapist rather than towards a blank screen, mirroring the treatment itself and not just early-life sediments. Therapy ceases to be exclusively a top-down process in which expert examines client through global protocols. It is unique to that patient and that analyst. The clinical experience can be seen as an intersubjective, third personality that mediates and, within its specific terms, incorporates, the two poles of the therapeutic dyad (Ogden, 1999). A relational therapist concisely captures the distance covered by the American school from its British predecessor by writing that 'Fairbairn was a one-person theorist': while sharing many of Fairbairn's premises, relational theory is dialogic, placing a social unit, a dyad, rather than an individual patient, as its main point of reference (Davies, 2004: 722).

Benjamin positions her work within this movement. For her, the dialogical content of the relational approach was implicit in psychoanalysis from its inception and thereby gains a teleological significance: it is the emerging truth of the discipline. Branching out from a physiological medicine that experimented with manipulating patients through hypnosis, late nineteenth-century Austrian psychoanalysis gradually learned that patients can be accessed through conversation. While the analyst was still the model-wielding professional, the patients' expression of their own thoughts became important. Acknowledging the significance of attachment and relating, midcentury object relations theory introduced these ingredients into the theory of how the psyche forms. The late-century relational approach advances beyond this point by subjecting therapeutic practice itself to the consequences of the theory: the value of the analytic process resides in its being a conversation between two subjects rather than in being an examination of a patient by an expert (Benjamin, 1998: 1–34). In the clinic, a composite existence surfaces that includes the two separate subjectivities of analyst and patient, *and* their shared, mutually attuned responses. This does not mean that within the clinical setting sociology takes over from psychology to condition an impassive subjectivity. On the contrary, the tensions and antagonisms explored within the dialogue manifest subjectivity's desire to assert itself against such conditioning, as the conversation goes through several defensive, aggressive and communicative modes. '[T]he analytic relationship', Benjamin (1998: 107) writes, 'provides some experience with the kind of intersubjective space that allows us to use identification to bridge difference, to hold multiple positions, to tolerate nonidentity rather than wipe out the position of self and other'.

Benjamin (1988: 42) places particular emphasis on differences and tensions. The therapeutic process corresponds to Winnicott's account of early differentiation. The child is not simply delivered from the agony of a formless internal world by the mother's reassuring consistency. Instead, the child has to destroy the mother so that she can survive and be acknowledged as a different individual who is not part of the child's interior

(Benjamin, 2018: 4). This is mirrored in the therapeutic setting where the analyst receives the patient's inputs, endures the discomfort caused by these inputs and connects the patient's distinct and unique individuality to another, similarly distinct but relating person (Gerhardt, Sweetnam and Borton, 2000). Benjamin (1988: 31–32) notes that in philosophical terms, the process corresponds to the Hegelian dialectic where, to gain a sense of its own humanity, the self seeks validation through a conflict that expresses the other's ability to resist, and through that resistance validate its own independent subjectivity. The turn to Hegel represents a change in the metaphysics at the background of psychoanalysis away from the Kantian, subject-object polarity that informed Freud's platform. In the relational approach as described and endorsed by Benjamin, the subject can no longer be grasped without another subject who responds to it. The meeting between the two pits thesis against antithesis to generate a third, synthetic option that allows room for both its constituents.

Gender Duality as Illness

Benjamin, then, deploys the insights of the relational school as a way of elaborating object relations theory. The third, intersubjective position that involves two mutually impacting individuals emerges in the clinic. Its triangulating perspective is the vehicle of therapy, which functions this way because it echoes and substitutes a healthy holding pattern that the home allows when it is allowed to function. If this is so, then the main disruption involves the inability to relate to another, independent subject. The child cannot conceive of the parent as a whole other who is both like the self and placed beyond the self's control. For Benjamin, the chief cause of this distortion is the society-wide construction of gender as a hierarchy.

The first, universal need of all children is the caring, containing and validating company of another human, usually a mother (Benjamin, 1988: 11–20). The mother holds the child's body, contains the child's changing states and names emotions, thus providing the child with the ability to self-regulate in a consistent way. This sets the platform for a coherent, reflexive individuality. For it to mature, the child has to perceive the mother as independent from the child's own being. Otherwise, the sense of individual distinction cannot be fully gained, while the modulation of feelings does not achieve the assuring resonance that can only come from outside one's own being. Individual agency and distinction, then, depend on letting go of the control wielded in fantasy over the parent. Benjamin relies on Margaret Mahler's study of child growth to flesh out how this potentiality unfolds within the timeline of motoric development. By the second year of life, spatial mobility is practised, and its experience is imbibed, teaching the child that distance from the mother can be created, extended and closed. The mother remains herself even when the child does not see her. When this insight is superimposed on Winnicott's notion of the object's destruction and survival, the result is that the distinction between self and other can be established alongside the realization that the other is trustworthy as an independent entity because she exists beyond the self's control. The ability to assess external reality, reason about it and tackle its constraints similarly develops by initially accepting the mother as both different from the self and like the self. The child produces an input. The mother responds with contents that differ from the child's, reflecting yet changing the child's input, thus handing over to the child a new perspective. They are looking at the same things and view them from differing positions that are valid because they are both subjects. In the process of exchanging such inputs, the child gains increasing abilities to process and order stimuli, thereby growing into an agent who contains inputs rather than an object that is overwhelmed by them. The nursing dyad consists of 'two active subjects [who] may exchange, may alternate in expressing and receiving, cocreating a mutuality that allows for and presumes separateness' (Benjamin, 1998: 29). The experience is emotionally rewarding as well as instrumentally empowering. Hence, in health, children not only tolerate, but cherish the independence of the other person as a corollary of that person's being relatable, and as enabling the self's own autonomy. One is an individual because one relates to other individuals, not despite that relationship (Benjamin, 1988: 30–34).

In health, children acquire the ability to distinguish genders late at this stage of differentiation. Consequently, Benjamin (1988) argues, gender does not have to disrupt or alter the link between individually distinct personhood and the recognition that others are similarly distinct and independent subjects. The oedipal father takes nothing substantial from a child who has relinquished phantasmic control over the mother. The reality principle has been tested, endured and accepted before Oedipus appears (40–41). The encounter with the father does not induce the fear that mutates into identification with and reverence for his supposed power. Nor does the mother appear weak by comparison. She is a person in her own right, so that the father does not contrast with a passive, homebound female. As the mother has already been released from close coexistence with the child through processes that are internal to healthy growth, the father holds no promise of delivering the child from a suffocating fusion with her. Gender does not appear as a differential in power or agency, and its terms do not contrast self-determining male with a dependent female. Moreover, the healthy development that proceeds through differentiation from the mother and the rapprochement with her as an independent person grants the child the ability to tolerate and partially resolve apparently opposing terms. I and other are not continuous as in omnipotent illusion, but they need not be mutually exclusive. Perception is not restricted to two exclusive options. As gender does not bear the weight of opposed sexual identities and is not fed into a perception structured by rigid dualities, it is internalized as relatively fluid (130–132). Boys can cross-identify with mothers who are perceived as fully human and therefore as akin to the subjectivity of their sons. Girls can take a matching, cross-identifying masculine perspective. Gender is another, negotiable dimension of individuality rather than one fixed identity out of two possible ones.

When gender does appear as a constraining duality, Benjamin argues, this arises from a configuration of the household that reciprocally conditions the broader social setting. When the mother is experienced as weak and dependent, the entire dynamic of growth takes on a different streak. Compared to the often-absent, distant and apparently freely travelling father, the mother seems a manipulable object. She cannot be a satisfactory source of validation, as she is not fully a real person. Such validation can only emanate from the powerful father. Autonomy is dislodged from the child's ability to relinquish control and relate to an essentially equal other. Instead, it attaches to the expectation of approval from a superior. The self-other differentiation is compromised by power, as the other is either dependent and inferior to the self, or wholly independent and superior to the self. As the gender distinction follows closely on the I-other distinction botched by the impact of polar hierarchy, hierarchic gender both compensates for the earlier distinction's failure and colours that distinction by creating two polarized sexual identities, only one of which is available to each person. Boys identify with the independent father. The oedipal phase becomes traumatic as it means giving up on one's closeness to the mother, generating the landscape accounted for by Freud. Girls align with the perceived abjectness of the mother (Benjamin, 1988: 100–107).

The gender hierarchy is replicated through individual subjectivity, along with the perception of the other as either an inferior to be controlled or a master to be feared. The duality permeates society and reproduces itself through various channels. The economic competition cultivated by capitalism divides the tasks related to the maintenance of the family and therefore encourages unequal parenting, keeping one parent closer to home while allowing the other a perceived freedom of movement and a liberating connection to the broader world. Media, educational institutions, literature and even the marketing of goods such as clothes and children's toys amplify representations of caring and emotion as opposed to hard-headed, independent agency. Sexuality is constructed and disseminated as involving the pursuit of a weaker object or the enticement of a stronger one. These various transmission routes reinforce each other. They are so prevalent that when one of them is hindered, for example by the spread of more egalitarian parenting norms, the others compensate for it to preserve gender as a dual hierarchy (Benjamin, 1988: 217–218).

The gender polarity is harmful because it disrupts the synergy of differentiation and relating. Casting the mother as passive and consequently structuring all relationships as hierarchies, the gender opposition hinders an existing human capacity: 'Polarity, the conflict of opposites, replaces the balance within the self' (Benjamin, 1988: 50). This extracts prices from individual and society alike. For individuals, neuroses are the outcome, as the relating that is the personality's core motivation finds no outlet in a validated and validating other, and is forced into the assertion of domination or the acceptance of subjection. On the societal level, gender polarity encourages the endorsement of aggression as the instrument of self-realization and cultivates the normalization of competition, hostility and violence. An outlook takes hold according to which we are primarily enemies fighting each other over scarce resources, and can become peaceful and cooperative only when subjugated. As we compete for survival, we assess the world around us as matter to be exploited and as a danger to be feared. Reason and knowledge become equated with the capacity to measure and compare aspects of a dead material world. The desiring subject views the mute object 'objectively', as in the thinking advanced by Descartes and Kant. Having no will of its own, the object can be exploited ruthlessly for the thinking subject's interests. This logic perceives itself as the opposite of caring, emotion and empathy with the environment: these are the attributes of the passive, feminine, sentimental and not-wholly-differentiated constituent (Benjamin, 1988: 189–198). An entire set of fixed and opposing pairs that are hierarchically ordered emerges, where masculine equals independent, active, ascendant, rational and emotionally detached, while feminine equals dependent, passive, submissive and governed by emotions to the exclusion of having independent discretion. As they are mutually excluding, these positions do not allow movement. No third position emerges to enable creativity and freedom.

Hegel, Feminism and Liberty

This critical assessment complements Benjamin's affirmative view of maternal agency, resulting in a comprehensive, descriptive and normative, account of both individual mind and collective dynamics. Before proceeding to examine this theory's implications for the notions of political freedom, democracy and liberalism, I would like to point out that Benjamin's outlook enables the mutual correction of several social approaches, thus pointing to the potentially far-reaching implications of object relations theory itself. Benjamin's deployment of object relations insights is capable of resolving issues that trouble the conceptual interface between psychoanalysis, feminist theory and Hegelian philosophy. It can account for the apparent anomaly that gender constitutes in Hegel's dialectic, it can shore up an affirmative ideal for psychoanalytical feminism and it can restructure dialectic in its entirety around gender. These issues are intertwined.

When laying down the groundwork for what will become second-wave feminism, Simone de Beauvoir (1989) argued that gender is an outlier in Hegel's dialectic. In every other relationship Hegel describes, the possibility for the self of being confirmed by the other involves admitting the other's independence and agency as a subject, which is conditioned on meeting that other's resistance as evidence of their independence. Collectivities gain political agency and enter history by organizing to resist, thus presenting an antithesis that the dominant thesis must confront, and so recognize. This is the case for nationalities, classes and cultures. But, de Beauvoir pointed out, not for genders. In the heterosexual bond, validation is given by someone who is essentially different from the self. Women do not collectively resist masculine domination because being a human female is the one identity that thrives on, rather than resists, another's ascendancy. No antithesis forms. Hierarchy reifies. Dialectic stalls in gender, while continuing to unfold elsewhere. For de Beauvoir, this meant that gender cannot be reduced to other hierarchies. It does not respond to the principles of any other relationship. Women's status cannot be essentially salvaged by reforms that address constitutional, legal or economic inequalities. It requires its own theory and its own activism, thereby necessitating the emergence of feminism as an independent approach.

De Beauvoir's account leaves open the question of why gender froze in this way, placing a constitutive human relationship beyond the logic of all other relationships. Attempts to answer this question in the decades following de Beauvoir's intervention resulted in different etiological and functional explanations ranging from the division of parenting tasks to the essence of what counts as heterosexual desire (MacKinnon, 1989; Okin, 1989). Alongside these explanations, a psychoanalytical one that associated with object relations and relational ideas was also proposed by such authors as Chodorow (1978) and Dinnerstein (1976). The internalized first relationship determines one's attitude to society. If that relationship's partner is a weakened woman, the gender hierarchy is perpetuated through the parental imagoes. Where society as a whole is patriarchal, the autonomy of the subject and the independence of the other are undermined by the mother's perceived dependence on the father, leading to an equation between femininity and submissiveness, and setting off the subsequent eroticization of power differentials that then presents itself as the normal form of desire. The fusion of feminist and object relations perspectives, then, augmented de Beauvoir's initial account by adding an explanation of how gender is accepted as a self-evident hierarchy. Chodorow (1991: 86–87) describes the deployment of psychoanalysis within feminist enquiry as primarily a critical tool that exposes the ways in which inequality is perpetuated within a formally egalitarian society.

Critics, however, alleged that object relations feminism lacked positive content and therefore propagated what it wanted to demolish: if gender is a codification of women's inferiority as transmitted and constructed by each individual psyche, then the only identity open to women as such is that weakness. The theory, it seemed to its detractors, found it difficult to conceive of an affirmative, empowering alternative that would process psychoanalytical insights into a feminist theory that has an operational, positive agenda (Hockmeyer, 1988).

Drawing on Winnicott, Benjamin (1988) provides object relations feminism with a positive ideal. Childcare can generate a tolerant, accepting and emotionally engaged egalitarianism. When the child accepts the mother as another person who can share, reflect and modify the child's perspective, the potentiality is generated of transcending 'the oppositions between powerful and helpless, active and passive' (48). Gender duality disrupts this potential, leaving the self to grapple with the binary of domination and passivity which invades all other social relations. Everyone is conditioned to fit into one of two complementary roles, and is accordingly confined by the limits of that role. Freedom and closeness alike 'become implicated in control and submission' (84). Political theories that accept violent power as their point of departure normalize illness rather than name valid principles for social organization. As psychoanalysis is rooted in its surrounding society, it, too, is implicated in these pathologies. Perspectives such as those of Thomas Hobbes found their way into Freud's casting of repression as the only way to control an ever-seething unconscious (3–5). Since Freud's account conveys the distortions of gender rather than a universally given condition, then repression and the ensuing neuroses need not be accepted as inevitable. Beyond them, the possibility of a healthier individuality and more egalitarian society can be glimpsed. In the form suggested by Benjamin, the alliance between feminism and object relations theory traces the outline for these possibilities, thus not only explaining how the dialectic skipped gender relations, but also furnishing feminism with a vision of an alternative societal order, while recognizing the special, historical and ongoing, role of women as primary parents.

Benjamin's combination of relations-based psychoanalysis and feminism also impacts on the political conclusions that can be derived from the concept of dialectic. Hegel thinks that our primary motivation is each self's will to be recognized as be an autonomous whole. As validation can only come from another subject who has similar wishes, it involves the admission that we cannot be absolute wholes. Every time we are rewardingly recognized, we sacrifice something. Every bond formed by such sacrifice immediately sets out on being recognized by the world outside it, thus requiring further losses. Conjugal partners combine into a bigger unit that now stands for the acting whole. By dividing their tasks between a homemaker and a breadwinner the partners grant a practical form to the requirement of sacrifice: none of them is an absolute. As households become synthetic subjects who also desire recognition, they combine into further groupings, cumulating in the state. As a final unit, the state is a whole that divides its tasks internally while representing the entire society to an outside world where no further synthetic level of organization exists. The relations of states are ultimately resolved by force, making politics a violent and coercive venture. The state's sovereignty stands for the subject's wish for solipsistic wholeness while enabling the lives of interrelating and differentiated individuals within it. Since the state appears as uncontested lethal power, participating in its life requires a different rationale than the life-affirming rationale of the home. Civic participation demands distance from our particular attachments, while the family demands commitment to these same attachments. For the state to exist, the family as the preserve of women needs to exist as well, but it needs to occupy a suppressed position whose rationale is barred from the surface of public life (Brooks, 2007).

Hegel, therefore, assumes that the price of recognition is the persistence of inequality and violence. This is one main reason for the hostility that liberals in the English-speaking world displayed towards Hegel. While they could concur with his emphasis on recognition as a constituent of individual autonomy, liberal thinkers preferred when pressed to fall back on the highly individualist and contractual perception of liberty offered by Locke and Mill: social validation was valuable, but the legal entitlements that protect us from each other and from government came first (Bradley, 1979; Franco, 1997). Paradoxically, when viewed from Benjamin's perspective, such reactions perpetuate whatever these liberals disliked about Hegel. Their upshot is to frame individual liberty as the ability to assert one's will unopposed in a specific area defined by rights and law, a notion that echoes the Hegelian subject's wish to be an unopposed absolute. Hence, individualist liberalism's attempt to resist Hegel falters, as seen in the recurring discomfort with the alienation, lack of solidarity, and paucity of communal venues often expressed by thinkers who attempt to reform liberalism from within. Object relations theory, however, may mend these faults. It frames the possibility of being a self-determining subject as something that occurs through an interaction that affirms peaceful egalitarianism rather than scuttles it. Benjamin (1988: 68–74) emphasizes Winnicott's contribution in particular. His model allows a validation process that does not lead to the assertion of absolute wholes against each other. The child destroys the mother, the mother survives to recognize the child, while the child acknowledges that psychic interiors contain the apparent contradictions of love and hate. We become autonomous not by declaring our unopposed sovereignty, but by tolerating and even welcoming the tension of different internal constituents alongside our acknowledgement of other subjects. Play allows pressing our superiority in one place, while admitting our dependence on others in other arenas and still acknowledging and valuing our fundamental, human equality. As we are bigger than any game we play, so is our play partner, who can accordingly survive our confrontational moves and our self-assertion within the game. If individuality ceases to be equated with an absolute and internally seamless form of agency, then no ultimate institutional authority is required to embody such agency. Individuals do not have to combatively assert themselves against each other, while the state does not have to stand for an unassailable totality that subjugates its citizens while fighting other states. Dialectic does not lead exclusively to oppression and war.

Moreover, if, when developing separately, object relations thought and feminist theory have benefited from Hegelian insights, then when brought together as Benjamin (1998: 100–101) suggests, they expose the limits of Hegel's worldview, and the places where that worldview may be opened up to other theoretical spaces. De Beauvoir had thought that gender was an outlier to a competitive dynamic that pervades all other social sites, but Benjamin's combination of psychoanalytic and feminist theory exposes gender as the origin of that dynamic. Growing up where the gender duality predominates teaches people that independence means assertive superiority over others, and that it contrasts with empathy, identification and fluidity. The ideal of selfhood equates with a rigid posture that treats any difference as a target for subjugation. The meeting of such selves plays out in conflict and ends with one of them submitting. The gender hierarchy is therefore the template of domination and subjection that becomes the struggle Hegel thinks is universal and inevitable. Gender survives the upheaval that dialectic brings to all other social sites because it is the dialectic's original platform. If this is granted, then Hegel's insight about the quest for validation can be endorsed without the attending baggage of inevitable conflict. We can concede the crucial role of the need for an object to relate to while keeping our ideals of liberty and equality. The coercion, oppression and war that liberals ascribed to Hegelian dialectic are consequences of its gendered character rather than ramifications of its fundamentally correct emphasis on recognition.

Benjamin, then, develops object relations theory by using the insights of the relational school, and then deploys the ensuing synthetic model of healthy growth within a feminist theory of mind and society. That theory covers not only issues that object relations theory itself neglected, such as the significance of the mother's subjectivity and agency, but also lacunas in the literature Benjamin brings in to address these issues, such as Hegelian philosophy and its feminist interpretation.

The Changing Grounds of Liberal Democracy

Beyond mediating these discrepancies within and among social philosophies, Benjamin's psychoanalytic model grounds its own positive, agenda-setting political theory. Like the object relations perspective on which it is based, this theory shares some key aspects with the historical manifestations of liberalism. Benjamin upholds individual freedom as an end and proposes a variant of natural law as a framework within which personal liberty can be made viable. Based on Winnicott's idea of transition and play, Benjamin frames the intersubjective meeting as a place where the partners conjointly create possibilities that were not available to them separately. Each player introduces a new move, to which the other has to accommodate by modifying their moves. The exchange ushers both participants into a new reality within the game's setting: by allowing agency to each participant, play grants a sense of movement and growth to both (Benjamin, 1998: 26–27). While made free in the minimalist sense of being exempted from anyone else's discretion when initiating moves, play also instils the more affirmative notion of liberty as freedom to create and grow (Yeatman, 2014).

Creation and growth entail the fluidity of one's own identity. The range of potentialities enlarged by the intersubjective meeting extends the bounds of the self by enabling it to perceive the world from the other person's perspective. To recognize the other as a subject who can initiate their own moves, the self has to imagine the other's point of view. The foundations for this capacity are put in place alongside the capacity to play itself. While waiting for the mother to return, the child who already holds an internalized representation of the mother can both retain a separate identity that is not threatened by the mother's absence, and identify with her as another person who has feelings and concerns like those of the self. One can leave and be left, be the caring adult and the cared-for child (Benjamin, 1999: 194). Identity can become flexible without endangering the viability of the individual subject. Freedom is enlarged by accepting the alterity of the other while valuing the other's presence and being capable of identifying with her. The acceptance of our relativity and incompleteness and the realization that the other is a subject like us 'makes multiple positions possible: not precisely identifying with all positions at once, but aware of their possibility' (Benjamin, 1998: 33). Intersubjectivity, therefore, enables liberty in the multiple senses of having discretion over our decisions, of enhancing our ability to move and create, and of enjoying the freedom to become different. These capacities reflect the concerns of various liberal theories with bolstering the space available for each person within the social order.

In addition to its attention to the rich meanings of personal liberty, Benjamin's theory advances a notion of impartial, universal and fair law that overrides positive legislation. This perception of law is related to the notion of freedom it protects. If personal freedom becomes viable within a setting where self and other are both distinct and interdependent, then asserting that freedom does not necessarily depend on policing by an external power. The intersubjective meeting can regulate itself, as both partners find the exchange with a similarly free and distinct other reassuring and conducive to their own sense of freedom. When the self allows the other to be different, that difference provides a validation of the self's own realness (Benjamin, 2018: 6). The potentiality for such combined agency and relating is shared by all, as it is rooted in early growth, making it a universally human feature. The internal regulation that takes place in the space where independent and mutually acknowledging subjects engage is accordingly also universal. Free and healthy subjects can generate a social existence in which all subjectivities can be accommodated, establishing a system of substantial, as opposed to positive, law. The intersubjective space that opens up between free individuals occupies in Benjamin's scheme an analogous position to that of the state of nature in Locke's. It is the site where people peacefully accommodate to each other by applying a system of understandings that are in principle global and inalienable from being human. Consequently, while valuing the plurality of opinions, experiences and cultures, Benjamin rejects a wholly relativist position of morality and law. Unless we retain a minimal perception of the humanity we share, the other's being different from us ceases to engage or challenge us and is not sensed as a source of validation (Benjamin, 1998: 101–104, 2018: 17).

The theory therefore entails subjecting positive law and the institutions that enforce it to criteria that precede them in the ethical and natural order. Law cannot be arbitrary or one-sided, or it would cease to be law and become a simple command that represents the whim of whoever utters it. Law cannot equate with the aggregation of specific, written laws formulated by legislatures and enacted by executives. Such positive legislation originates in a specific centre, such as a parliament, which presupposes a state and its borders. Its stipulations aspire to be interlocking, so as to minimize internal contradictions. For the same reason, such legislation applies to all citizens. Accordingly, positive legislation is essentially a single will that proceeds according to its own logic and obligates its subjects regardless of circumstances and identities. Unless bound by more universal, ethical guidelines that transcend specific institutions, positive legislation is arbitrary. In its fundamental, inclusive and respectful sense, by contrast, law emanates from the interpersonal processes of recognition, tension and the containment of tension that underlie individual liberty itself. The intersubjective meeting in which real, natural law is grounded should shape actual public bodies: 'The function of the Third – representing a lawful world in which more than one can live – needs to be socially embodied in genuinely protective social institutions' (Benjamin, 2018: 247). By valuing a notion of individual liberty that has a social aspect derived from the first experiences, and by linking this liberty to a universal, natural and morally obliging law, Benjamin echoes fundamental liberal concepts.

However, by placing these ingredients in a structure informed by the amalgamation of object relations thought and feminist theory, Benjamin also differs from the canonical forms of liberal philosophy, as in Locke or Mill. Primarily, this can be seen in her argument that groups, as well as individuals, should ideally participate in the process of generating new perspectives by enabling mutual recognition. Communities and cultures are the environments where individuals meet as particular humans who can engage within a reasonably familiar setting, echoing the potentialities of the original, mother-child encounter. The meeting between these communities replicates the dynamics of the meeting between individual selves. It confronts every group identity with another actor who is like the self and therefore elicits empathic interest and identification, and is yet different enough to challenge the self. The encounter prompts a process by which communities validate each other's experience, vulnerability and legitimacy. Communities whose experiences include persecution and discrimination may become entitled to compensation as a measure of such reciprocal collective recognition. This is required not only for bolstering these communities, but for offering a concrete venue through which the other, hurt-inflicting communities can recognize their own conflicted baggage, a process that echoes Winnicott's notion of concern and reparation (Benjamin, 1998: 91–92). To enable liberty, then, rights and law should foster the individual's capacity to engage with others, the arenas where that engagement takes place and the space between these arenas. This makes for a move beyond liberalism's traditional emphasis on individuals as the primary units of the social order and on their role as the subjects of rights.

The implications of Benjamin's stand on the role of groups exceed the simple extension of the rights previously accorded to individuals, to groups. Contemporary political philosophers have worked to reconcile liberalism and community by supplementing individual rights with the entitlement to belong communally and the entitlement to freely express that sense of belonging. This effort to extend the content of rights can be thought of as the next logical step after the welfare state: individuals merit rights to life, liberty and property, as in classical liberalism; rights to education and health services as in welfare liberalism; and rights to communal life and collective recognition, as in the late twentieth-century communitarian interpretation of liberalism (Benhabib, 2011; Kymlicka, 2001). Additionally, this line of thought borrows insights from the pluralist variants of historical liberalism by demanding that the groups themselves be granted entitlements and recognition as legal bodies, so as to be better able to represent and shield their constituents (Levy, 2015). The resulting social order is a network of social enclaves protected from each other as individuals are shielded from intrusion by the constitutional rights to life, liberty and welfare. Liberalism accommodates itself to a more complex, postmodern society while remaining nonetheless true to its core beliefs.

Benjamin (1998: 101–102) does not necessarily adhere to this view. She warns that implementing such agendas would isolate worldviews from each other. If groups are shielded from interference and individuals are seen as best protected and enabled when living within such groups, then the danger lurks that each person would meet only with the like-minded, limiting venues for significant dialogue. If the self is not challenged by inputs that originate in a differing subjectivity, it can neither healthily differentiate nor gain a fulfilling source of validation. Moreover, adding cultural and communal rights to the individualist package of entitlements requires naming specific addressees to whom such rights can be imputed, ascribing a fixed identity and a seamless cohesion to each group. But if communal identities are like individual ones, then they, too, are neither seamless nor fixed. Establishing them as known identities would encourage them to close ranks, flaunt their supposed unity, snuff out internal difference and limit communication with an outside that would be presented in the paranoid-schizoid terms of an alien threat. Communal relations will become a series of grudge-affirming demands (Benjamin, 2018: 238). For Benjamin, such a result is harmful. If the self is to be productively impacted by recognizing the other's subjectivity, and if the self is to acknowledge the hurt it has inflicted and take responsibility for its own multiplex interior, it has to do so voluntarily: the process is at bottom a psychological one, providing a common thread to 'early individual repair and later reparation of social injustice' (Benjamin, 2018: 246). If imposed by law and government, expressions of concern and regret might trigger an inward turn by the perpetrators, who would focus on their own grievances and their own identity rather than fruitfully converse (Benjamin, 2018: 237–240, 247). Imagining social relations, and then politics and law, in terms of rights and entitlements modelled on the rights held by the detached individual of classical liberalism is for Benjamin an error that perpetuates the errors of that liberalism. Its hub is to perceive identities as mutually isolated rather than as communicating and mutually forming.

Instead of attempting to correct this mechanic form of individualism by borrowing its terms for the use of groups, Benjamin expects freely expressed collective affiliations to challenge the very notion of rights as exclusive properties. As with individual subjects, the life of collective identities should be understood through the lens of what happens in the first bond. When the mother reappears after the child's attack on her, she illustrates for the child the possibility of withstanding destruction. As a real and whole person, she acknowledges the child's emotions, deploying symbolization and language to help the child make sense of feelings. These acts establish the relating, active presence of another person as synergetic with individuation (Benjamin, 1998: 29). Holding allows the mother to safely and even productively err. When she misnames the child's feelings, the mother establishes herself as both close to the child, as she communicates her perceptions to the child, and different from the child, as she errs when presenting the child's state. The good achieved by this outweighs the pain of misunderstanding, rendering children capable of tolerating 'a fair amount of the misattunement that is intrinsic to relating to another' (Benjamin, 2000: 49). In the clinic, this insight informs the therapist's effort to reflect the patient's state, both as an expression of recognition and as an attempt to process experience. The clinician might miss the mark in terms of content, but the act of striving to reflect the patient back more than compensates for the error as it confirms the legitimacy of the patient's interior and furnishes the patient with an instance of a different, flawed subjectivity (Benjamin, 1998: 25). The experience of misrecognition is an aspect of the overall pattern of conflict and survival: the child cannot destroy the mother in fantasy, the mother cannot destroy the child with words. They both return to the interaction as two autonomous subjects.

In a similar way, groups and cultures are shaped by encountering other collectives, whose initial reactions are understandably off the mark in terms of each group's experience of its own life. The dialectic pressure of an initially alien perspective induces a recognition of that perspective, at first expressed as disbelief and criticism, but then taking the form of the wish to understand, which is mutually reinforced by the corresponding efforts of the other group. While misrecognition and false closure might trigger resentment, they also enable an ultimately fruitful sequence of breakdown and reparation that echoes the destruction and reconciliation cycle of the child's differentiation (Benjamin, 1998: 97). Each collectivity is enriched by the indeterminate, tense moments of the interaction. Difference is valued rather than suppressed. All actors are invested in maintaining diversity and accordingly do not aspire to control others, mould them in their own image, or even internally impose a closured, fixed perception of the group's own identity (Benjamin, 1998: xx). As the social order that enables and is, in turn, constituted by such encounters generates the possibility of mutual recognition, it does not have to be coercive: it is essentially democratic. The natural law that governs relationships between mutually recognizing subjects is not overridden by positive law. Public life can become a space for communication rather than primarily an arena for existential struggles, legalist argumentation and haggling over scarce resources. Instead of public indifference to our particular identities, the shared societal life envisioned by Benjamin allows these identities to be acknowledged and mediated. The resulting social landscape does not easily equate with the individualist liberal vision, or even with what is entailed by liberalism's pluralist and communitarian modes. The dynamic of the first relationship where the child's sense of self is given tolerable coherence by engagement with the parent extends into the public sphere to push back the rigid language of legislation and fixed entitlements.

Benjamin, then, endorses the value of individual autonomy upheld by liberalism as well as proposes a form of natural society and natural law that resemble those adopted by historical liberalism. However, she modifies liberalism's perceptions of rights and the spheres where they operate.

Rather than prioritizing a politics that plays out within specialized spaces such as elections, parliaments and magistracies, she emphasizes a dialogue that replicates and extends the intersubjective encounter of parent and child. As a result, Benjamin populates what would have been the civic side of the sphere division with dynamics that reflect the original, supposedly private, meeting of self and world. Benjamin thus offers a political theory that takes into account both the insights of relational psychoanalysis and the concerns of the late-century setting: the awareness of constitutional democracy's limits, and the understanding that truth and knowledge develop through a tense conversation between different positions rather than constitute a given, interlocking system. Rather than a top-down imposition of unified law and knowledge, Benjamin envisions a series of encounters between individuals and groups who challenge each other's perceptions as well as their own. It is a world in which self and other, subjectivity and objectivity are not sharply opposed, and correspondingly avoid the replication of the gender polarity and its attending hierarchy.

Persistent Dualism

However, Benjamin's reliance on object relations models in which the holding environment is the bedrock of healthy relating and individuality alike involves a certain difficulty. As Benjamin intentionally lowers the partition between privacy and politics, she imports the duality of the holding situation itself into what should have been a strictly egalitarian arena for collective decision.

Locke separated the spheres as a move against contemporary apologias for absolutism which cast the king as the father of his people. In these apologias, submission to a superior who is stronger than us, knows better than us and cares for us, was framed as inborn and intuitive. Negating it contradicts our most basic experiences: if one demands rights to hold against the king, then one has to accept the absurdity of a dependent child demanding entitlements against the providing and protecting parent. Locke's counter-argument was that parental authority is limited in essence. Parents care for their children as long as they actually are children, and can expect obedience as a necessary condition of performing such guardianship. But parents do not have the power of life and death over their children, as that would contradict their task of seeing their children safely into adulthood along with the authority that this task temporarily grants them. Grownup offspring cease to be their parents' dependents and can only be governed by consent, which also invokes responsibility to law and accountability to its penalties. From Locke's point of view, then, insistence on the continuity of home and politics is wrong, as it confuses the realm of dependence and guardianship with that of responsibility and law (Locke, 1946).

Benjamin's perception may seem immune to such risks, as the initial bond she describes establishes mutual recognition between independent subjects: there is no archaic, predetermined sphere where everything follows from animal functions. In health, we are within a sphere of rational, differentiated and essentially equal agents from the very start. While the mother appears as a provider and the child as a supplicant, the recognition of the mother as another person allows imagining the reversal of roles through imagination and play. The form of play itself induces the notion 'that both partners are equal' (Benjamin, 1988: 48). The mutual respect for others as differing from the self and meriting spaces where they exercise their own discretion is acquired in the first bond. The basis for the norms of equality, impartiality and individual autonomy that underlie constitutional law are internalized within the private sphere. A public life characterized by equality and the autonomy of each person is predicated upon a healthy home life which is pervaded by similar values. The sphere distinction, itself a projection of patriarchal imagination, need not be insisted on.

But the supportive home environment Benjamin envisions still necessitates a caring parent and a dependent child as its premise. The complementary duality has to be there first and furnish the ground on which the egalitarian potentiality can unfold. Benjamin realizes that the nursing dyad involves a powerful, yet accountable, provider, and a weaker partner who is initially absolved from responsibility. The clinical setting mimics this relationship with therapist and patient (Benjamin, 2000: 46). In both cases, the liberation of the subject into full agency and a matching capacity for recognition depends on a differential in power and responsibility.

One consequence of this structure is that the parental role becomes more constraining for those who perform it. This may seem far from Benjamin's intention, as she emphasizes the mother's status as a real person who has her own concerns rather than being the abjectly selfless giver of patriarchal imagination (McKay, 2019). However, constrains on mothers are still implied. Some of them might be marginal to the scope of the theory. If the mother performs mechanically as a dutiful service-provider, she becomes a less-than-human object for her child. To avoid this, she has to apply will and thought, to constantly tap her emotional depth and skilfully confront the child with it in their interaction. She has to be present in the game, 'catching and throwing' rather receiving, collecting, or tidying up (Benjamin, 1998: 29). In the reality of childcare, this might imply a certain aggravation of parental burdens. To comply with the requirement of presenting their children with actively willing partners, parents have to suspend their own troubling concerns, their exhaustion, anxiety and boredom, and be, or at worst simulate, a lively presence when interacting with their children. This proviso might ground the call, popular in the final years of the twentieth century, for parents to spend 'quality time' with children (Hochschild, 1997). Benjamin (1988), to be sure, does not advise such an approach, as she is emphatic that parental exhaustion is disruptive for the healthy course of growth she describes (14, 24, 27–28). Her premises, however, can take this form when put into operative guidelines.

More substantially, for Benjamin, performing the parental role in a certain way is the condition for the entire social order. By suggesting an approach to society and politics that extends the dynamics of the home, Benjamin tasks the mother with preventing war that the sovereign is tasked with by Hobbes. For Hobbes, the need for recognition joins, rather than counters, material scarcity's tendency to propel chaos. In nature, humans seek what Hobbes calls glory, which is validation of their worth. As there is hardly any amiable interaction in nature, validation can only be extracted forcefully, leading to violence as a vehicle for achieving glory. Only the sovereign's superior force can grant humans the occasion to meaningfully communicate. This perception of conflict as following, not only on material scarcity but on the need for social validation, also informs Hegel's dialectic, as it does Freud's account of the oedipal situation. In all cases, relationships generate tensions and fears that require a superior agent to police them. In Benjamin's scheme, by contrast, parental holding can instil egalitarian respect, curiosity and the ability to cross-identify. These abilities pull the child out of the ever-lurking paranoid-schizoid mode, resulting in a world of communicating and free subjects who cherish each other's freedom as conducive to their own (Benjamin, 2018: 5–6). Differences are valued and the friction between them is non-violently negotiated rather than pressed until one side succumbs. Consequently, Benjamin (1999: 194) writes, 'power is dissolved'. The maternal agency central to Benjamin's theory aligns with an ascendant natural law that, as it pre-emptively resolves chaos, obviates the enforcing sovereign. The intersubjective encounter of child and parent that occupies in Benjamin's scheme the position that the benign state of nature occupies in Locke consists in 'two subjects regulating each other' rather than in 'one subject regulating another' (Benjamin, 1988: 45). Being in principle universal and achievable, this perception of maternal agency finalizes Locke's victory over Hobbes without resorting to the separation of spheres Locke advocates.

But this free society hinges on the performance of the parental role. Care may include agency, but the function of caring remains essential: all other positions and actions can be creatively developed, challenged and transformed, but that of a caregiver retains its universal features as all others depend on it. That role is one pole in a complementary duality, whose other pole is entitled to the ministrations of its partner because no dignified human life would be possible without it. Parenting as deliberate effort and agency is a plausible concept. However, parenting as agency that is equal to the child's within a conceptual framework that focuses on the child's development is less so, especially as the Kleinian basis in an initially disorganized infancy persists. The parent is a constant, primarily physical, presence, from which the cared-for child can venture forth into creativity. The child's ability to become a subject who is capable of recognizing the mother as another subject is made possible by '[t]he mother', acting 'as an outside other who is able to help the subject...process and tolerate internal states of tension' (Benjamin, 1998: 27). Her initial appearance is that of a concrete physical other, a body whose corporeal characters – breathing and tactile pressure – form the holding environment. The maternal body is the necessary starting point, the solid, incontestable ground on which the movement of speech and play may take place. The body is a person. Whatever her other capacities, her being there is her crucial activity. She is the axiom beyond which no further probing is possible. Transformative dialogue is rooted in something which is not dialogue and cannot be transformed.

Parent and child, therefore, constitute a duality in which one partner provides the stability on which the other's movement is predicated. Is their duality necessarily gendered? Is the mother necessarily female? Along with the egalitarian and responsive sharing of parental tasks, Benjamin encourages the ability to identify with the other without giving up on the self. Our identities need not be seen as fixed properties that are glued to anatomy. Benjamin (1988: 113) suggests that individuals 'should integrate and express both male and female aspects of selfhood'. However, Benjamin's scheme entails that this very ability to transcend strict binary divisions necessitates a prior division of holder and held. That division remains the single complementary binary in a world where all other identities are (ideally) negotiable. We may be able to identify as any gender, we may desire and be desired, we may leave or be left, but we cannot transcend container and contained. Women have performed as mothers historically and have been denigrated and marginalized for doing so, and Benjamin's theory demonstrates that they should instead be vindicated and empowered for it. If gender is understood as a complementary dual hierarchy, and if the role of mother, in the sense of the holding partner in the nursing dyad, is irreducible, then the one place where one can locate gender in the model Benjamin elaborates is motherhood. The correlation of the responsibility for the social order and the positioning of women in the role where that responsibility resides generates a special weight for women to shoulder: this Atlas cannot shrug. Her burden is everyone else's freedom.

The complementarity of holder and held has the further implication of nudging out the possibility of any space that legitimately and healthily refrains from replicating the holding dynamics. The mother attunes to the child's conduct and names the child's feelings until the child can do so independently. The therapist offers a human figure to identify with as the patient finds internal regulation difficult. The mother's or therapist's presence provide the platform on which the dynamic of destruction and survival play out, making error and misattunement beneficial rather than harmful. The relationship Benjamin (2000) describes is two-tiered: a secure basis guaranteed by the holding partner and an arena for differences to play out, in which the holding partner is treated as equal to the self. Made safe for the weaker, less secure partner, the setting is ready for the conversation that neutralizes weak and strong as it proceeds through a language which is accessible to all:

> nonverbal attunement creates the original space of thirdness in which the free-flowing back-and-forth does not appear as a reaction to the other's demand but as the partners' mutual creation of a dance—the first form of mutual recognition. This space later becomes that of dialogue, in which it becomes possible to create meanings that transcend those of the singular person and to analyze the interaction between two partners. It is here that negotiation of difference creates a different, more symbolic form of recognition.
>
> (49)

Throughout, the differences in power and stakes allow the parent or clinician to take the necessary risks. They can express confusion, anger, desire and desperation as illustrations of their vulnerable humanity, allowing the child or patient to identify with them and concede their own, comparable sensations. Such expressions do not endanger the positions of parent and analyst, because the functional differentiation of adult and child, paid professional and paying client, holder and held, assures these positions alongside the continuity of the relationship itself. The parent would still be stronger than, and responsible for, the child, if she shows vulnerability (Benjamin, 2000: 53). The dialectic is experienced as total for the junior party, but as limited for the senior one: the antithesis is anticipated, assumed and resolved in advance.

It is a feature of Benjamin's worldview that such a necessary differential in power relations cannot remain localized in parenting or therapy. The predication of adult behaviour on childhood experiences is premised by psychoanalysis itself, while the continuity between individual mind and society at large is a quality of object relations theory, where the mind is structured by the social environment and feeds back into it. The feminist literature on which Benjamin relies points to similar conclusions: roles, relationships and power differentials in the most intimate settings mutually reflect on the entire society. Moreover, Benjamin actively promotes such continuity between home and society as part of her normative agenda, since she views the sphere separation as an inflection of the gender hierarchy. The impersonal legal structures that supposedly characterize the traditional perception of the civic sphere 'express the primary course of gender domination' (Benjamin, 1988: 216). Consequently, Benjamin expects public dynamics to further elaborate the initial bond's process of mutual recognition, as that process goes through stages of strife, friction, misrecognition, breakdown and survival. 'Politically', she writes, 'the possibility of mutual intersubjectivity is predicated on the very difference that also leads to continual misfiring of recognition' (Benjamin, 1998: 101). If the rationale of early holding and its horizon of intersubjectivity are expected to impact politics as they do other sites, then the implication of a junior and senior partner on which the possibility of intersubjective communication depends attaches to politics as well. The formal equality of legal personas and civil rights depends on, and takes it cues from, another arena, where the participants are complementary. Benjamin thus both cultivates a perception of domesticity and politics as continuous, and proposes an unequal holding situation as the natural, underlying and healthy social bedrock.

Benjamin imagines a public arena where individuals and groups alike gain recognition and enrich their perceptions by engaging with the alterity of the other. However, where collective life-and-death decisions are taken and no external mediator exists, everyone is compelled to seek advantages and struggle to maintain them. Every utterance is potentially strategic and life-threatening: intersubjectivity breaks into the assertion of opposed, paranoid selves, all facing each other as threats. Expressions of internal content by individuals and groups, as in standing on one's specific cultural or historical identity, acquire the character of bargaining chips. The other parties would do their utmost to discount such claims rather than open-mindedly, if agonizingly, engage with them. Some agent, then, has to modulate if the spread of the Hobbesian pattern is to be prevented. Some observers understand Benjamin as suggesting that, as relationships in wider society are always made unequal by some advantage a participant has, then that participant should take the responsibility for holding and enabling the dialogue with the other participant. The stronger partner should contain its own hurt and anxiety so as to acknowledge, and ultimately allow for acknowledgement by, the other partner (Frosh, 2011). But if such a guideline seems morally appealing, Benjamin's own premises undermine it. In an authentic exchange that challenges our beliefs, we all should, as follows the dialectical nature of such communication, feel hurt, marginalized and endangered. Destruction and tension are essential for the process. 'In fact', Benjamin (1998: 85) writes, 'if the other were not a problem for the subject, the subject would again be absolute – either absolutely separate or assimilating the other'. In a setting where collective existential issues are at stake and where the relatively stronger partner's position cannot be assured, that partner has no guarantee of their own survival. Defences cannot be lowered and the other, supposedly weaker side, cannot be offered tolerance and recognition. Where nobody has lingering superiority, nobody can survive social conflict in the way that the conversing self 'survives' within a dialogue that takes place in the more structured setting of the family or the clinic.

Alford (1990) makes the point that beyond a certain size, human groups cannot maintain the level of trust that personal relations may allow. In a Kleinian model, this would activate the paranoid-schizoid position, and so consign politics to an existence where some level of violence cannot be avoided. However, in a democracy as conventionally understood, the same effect is generated by the strict egalitarianism of that polity's premises. If citizens who are made equal, and therefore equally vulnerable, by their formal entitlement cannot be counted on for holding the debate because the stakes are too high for them, who can take on the public-sphere role which is analogous to that of mother or therapist? Does it cohere with Benjamin's scheme if the responsible partner takes the form of a juristic system entrusted with interpreting the underlying, inclusive law, and so critique and maybe overturn the positive legislation made by the representatives of sparring vested interests? Or should we perceive educators, scholars, scientists and therapists as having the ability to observe social conflict from a triangulating perspective, and thus as qualified to limit the harm that the players might inflict on each other? That these questions are raised at all points to a background factor: if Benjamin's perspective is taken to its logical end, then politics, as the activity of formally equal agents deciding collectively on existential matters where no further instance is available for mediation, becomes extinct. It exists nowhere, as the whole range of social interactions is expected to be ideally inhabited by inflections of the original, holding situation.

Conclusion

Writing within the late-century setting of American relational thinking, Benjamin combines feminist, Hegelian and object relations insights. Using Winnicott's concepts, Benjamin stresses that the mother has to be experienced by the child as an independent subject with her own will and her own legitimate concerns. When the mother acts as an autonomous agent, the child can develop a sense of personhood within a context of two relating subjects. The process, however, is distorted when societal conditions intervene to present the mother as less than an independent person, dividing dependence and care from autonomy, female from male, archaic and 'natural' from rational and fully human. Consequently, the nourishing ability to communicate with others is hampered, breaking down into opposing contrasts. The tendency manifest in society, law, politics and scientific thought to split all fields into complementary and unequal dualisms such as self and other, subject and object, reason and intuition, follows from the damage wrought by imbibing opposed gender roles. To correct it, Benjamin offers to emphasize recognition through dialogue as a process that dialectically forms self and other alike. An egalitarian environment is crucial for such communication to take place, as dialogue allows movement and development for each person alongside the recognition of the other as a different and autonomous subject.

Benjamin's thought reconciles discrepancies within and among the various sources she deploys. They are all placed within a coherent descriptive and normative framework that has a political dimension. Benjamin's overriding concern is the autonomy, agency and dignity of each individual. She proposes weaving the social order around this concern. Benjamin similarly holds political institutions and positive legislation to the bar of a universal set of norms elaborated through the interactions of mutually recognizing humans. Her perception accordingly matches that of a constitutionalist and liberal approach to democracy.

At the same time, Benjamin's alliance with liberalism and democracy as conventionally understood is confined by her stated end of diminishing the boundary between privacy and politics, and by the related idea of the first bond's influence on later life. For Benjamin, the sphere division is another case of a polarizing and gendered terminology which pits complementary oppositions against each other. Accordingly, enabling public life to be more directly impacted by the dynamics acquired in the first bond is for her a valued end. When healthy, the nursing dyad allows the child to gain autonomy on the basis of holding. Difference, friction and even hostility do arise, but are utilized within the process for propelling autonomy and creativity. However, the first bond still involves a complementary duality. The mother's having responsibility over the child is the stable platform on which the more dynamic engagements rely. If the public world of civic and political participation is to be continuous with the empathy and relatedness of the home, then it becomes continuous with the home's founding hierarchy, which is based on the function women are historically identified with. Such a continuity also suggests that the public sphere itself should be structured by the greater responsibility, and implicitly, the broader perspective and ensuing authority, ascribed to some of its participants.

This outcome can be accounted for by the interventions of feminist theory and newly elaborated perceptions of knowledge and science. Benjamin uses these resources as responses to the challenges of the time and the concerns characteristic of the relational school's setting. By offering this worldview, Benjamin aims to cultivate a dialogue of different groups and cultures without privileging a centre, while still being committed to a shared, universally binding ethics. But her approach can also be seen as predicated on the trajectory of object relations thought when driven by its own, internal and professional concerns. By synthesizing Klein's two positions, Fairbairn's perception of humans as object seeking rather than gratification seeking, and Winnicott's notions of transition and play, Benjamin lands close to the vision offered by Ian Suttie and Jane Suttie 50 years earlier, grounding a comprehensive, social and political outlook in a specific psychoanalytical theory. This outlook includes a dynamic, expanding private sphere that evolves out of the relationship of mother and child to enfold society, until its formally political and civic space forfeits some of the distinctive function it was tasked with by older democratic thought.

References

Alford, C.S. (1990). Reparation and civilization: A Kleinian account of the large group. *Free Associations* 1T (19): 7–30.
Beauvoir, S. de (1989). *The second sex*. New York: Vintage.
Benhabib, S. (2011). *Dignity in adversity: Human rights in troubled times*. Cambridge: Polity.
Benjamin, J. (1988). *The bonds of love*. New York: Pantheon.
Benjamin, J. (1998). *Shadow of the object*. London: Routledge.
Benjamin, J. (1999). Recognition and destruction: An outline of intersubjectivity. In Mitchell, S.A., and Aron, L. (eds.), *Relational psychoanalysis: The emergence of a tradition*. Hillsdale, NJ: The Analytic Press, 181–210.
Benjamin, J. (2000). Intersubjective distinctions: Subjects and persons, recognitions and breakdowns. *Psychoanalytic Dialogues* 10 (1): 43–55.
Benjamin, J. (2018). *Beyond doer and done to*. New York: Routledge.
Berman, E. (1997). Relational psychoanalysis: A historical background. *American Journal of Psychotherapy* 51: 185–203.
Bradley, J. (1979). Hegel in Britain: A brief history of British commentary and attitudes. *The Heynthrop Journal* 20 (1): 1–24.
Brooks, T. (2007). *Hegel's political philosophy*. Edinburgh: Edinburgh University Press.
Chodorow, N. (1978). *The reproduction of mothering*. Berkeley: University of California Press.
Chodorow, N. (1991). *Feminism and psychoanalytic theory*. New Haven, CT: Yale University Press.
Davies, J.M. (2004). Whose bad objects are we anyway? Repetition and our elusive love affair with evil. *Psychoanalytic Dialogues* 14 (6): 711–732.
Dinnerstein, D. (1976). *The mermaid and the minotaur: Sexual arrangements and human malaise*. New York: Harper & Row.
Flax, J. (1981). Psychoanalysis and the philosophy of science: Critique or resistance? *The Journal of Philosophy* 78 (10): 561–569.
Flax, J. (1990). *Thinking fragments*. Berkeley and Los Angeles: University of California Press.
Franco, P. (1997). Hegel and liberalism. *The Review of Politics* 59 (4): 831–860.
Frosh, S. (2011). The relational ethics of conflict and identity. *Psychoanalysis, Culture and Society* 16: 225–243.
Gerhardt, J., Sweetnam, A., and Borton, L. (2000). The intersubjective turn in psychoanalysis: A comparison of contemporary theorists: Part 1: Jessica Benjamin. *Psychoanalytic Dialogues* 10 (1): 5–42.
Hale, N.G., Jr. (1995). *Freud in America* v. 2. Oxford: Oxford University Press.
Hochschild, A. 1997. *The time bind: When work becomes home and home becomes work*. New York: Henry Holt and Company.

Hockmeyer, A. (1988). Object relations theory and feminism: Strange bedfellows. *Frontiers: A Journal of Women Studies* 10 (1): 20–28.

Kymlicka, W. (2001). *Politics in the vernacular*. Oxford: Oxford University Press.

Lasch, C. (1984). *The minimal self*. New York: W.W. Norton.

Levy, J.T. (2015). *Rationalism, pluralism, and freedom*. Oxford: Oxford University Press.

Locke, J. (1946). *The second treatise of civil government*. Oxford: Basil Blackwell.

MacKinnon, C. (1989). *Toward a feminist theory of the state*. Cambridge, MA: Harvard University Press.

McKay, R.K. (2019). Where objects were, subjects now may be: The work of Jessica Benjamin and reimagining maternal subjectivity in transitional space. *Psychoanalytic Inquiry* 39 (2): 163–173.

Meehan, J. (2002). Arendt and the shadow of the other. *International Journal of Philosophical Studies* 10 (2): 183–193.

Mitchell, S.A. (2003). *Can love last?* New York: W.W. Norton.

Mitchell, S.A., and Aron, L. (1999). Preface. In Mitchell, S.A., and Aron, L. (eds.), *Relational psychoanalysis: The emergence of a tradition*. Hillsdale, NJ: The Analytic Press, ix–xx.

Ogden, T. (1999). The analytic third: Working with intersubjective analytical facts. In Mitchell, S.A., and Aron, L. (eds.), *Relational psychoanalysis: The emergence of a tradition*. Hillsdale, NJ: The Analytic Press, 459–492.

Okin, S.M. (1989). *Justice, gender, and the family*. New York: Basic.

Seligman, S. (2019). Relational psychoanalysis as a 'child of the sixties': Politics, innovation, and the transition from adolescence. *Psychoanalytic Inquiry* 39 (2): 146–155.

Westerman, M.A. (2005). What is interpersonal behavior? A post-Cartesian approach to problematic interpersonal patterns and psychotherapy process. *Review of General Psychology* 9 (1): 16–34.

Winnicott, D.W. (1984). *Through paediatrics to psychoanalysis*. London: Karnac.

Yeatman, A. (2014). A two-person conception of freedom: The significance of Jessica Benjamin's idea of intersubjectivity. *Journal of Classical Sociology* 15 (1): 3–23.

Conclusion

Object relations theory emerged alongside a certain range of new approaches in political philosophy and in the wider public discussion. The psychoanalytical theory mirrored some of these perspectives. In particular, the emphasis that authors like Ian Suttie, Fairbairn and Winnicott placed on parental care as a condition for the healthy autonomy of the adult individual matched welfare-state liberalism's perception of individual freedom as entailing planned and centralized, if limited, measures of governmental intervention in economy and society. The psychoanalysts similarly concurred with the advanced liberals' tendency to relax the division of the private sphere from politics by expecting the units that make up the private realm to become creative and dynamic, to a degree that impacts formally political, civic life. This tendency was shared by more midcentury ideologies than welfare-state liberalism.

With their patients zero being schizoids rather than hysterics, a turn described by Fairbairn, echoed by Winnicott, and finally and comprehensively recounted by Guntrip, object relations analysts trace illness to a deficiency of integration and to the splitting of personality levels into separate fields. The outcome of such splitting is that engagement with the outside, concrete world is faulty and vulnerable, while the secluded, internal components of the personality become depleted. Correspondingly, object relations analysts equate health with a layered and complex, but ultimately integrated, individual personality, for which engagement with society mutually enriches a sheltered internal life. The social order entailed by this analytical approach reflects the concept of individual integration and translates it to the societal level, allowing for a multi-layered and dynamic structure of society in which all modes of interaction benefit each other. Conversely, the concept of an autonomous, merely formalistic and jurisdictional realm of politics that is detached from other human concerns is cast as a society-wide variant of what on the individual level appears as a paranoid-schizoid propensity to split and project.

The health thus conceptualized is achieved by allowing a proper space for sociability. By substituting the child's wish to relate for Freud's sexualized libido and Klein's innate, destructive instinct, object relations analysts transformed the character of the primary bond into a naturally benevolent one. Organizational units that individuals create later in life can in principle follow on the patterns established by the primary bond, and may then similarly take place in a largely power-free space. While differences are tolerated and the necessity for negotiation – rather than the availability of immediate harmony – is recognized, the high-stake fight for survival that turns everything into a zero-sum engagement is excluded. Feminist critics took the analysts to task for reading power out of their concept of the home, thus placing its differentials outside political enquiry. But from the analysts' point of view, such an enquiry is redundant: assuming the operation of an irreducibly competitive and aggressive attitude that seeks to get even in all circumstances is itself a mark of illness that might be generated by the misplaced intervention of an external, non-natural world. Ian Suttie's child is left with no residual sense of resentment because attachment to the caring parent carries no cultural stigma and involves no shame. Winnicott's child converts aggression into a more complex attachment than the original mother-baby bond through the mother's survival and the ensuing ability to play. As destructive aggression need not arise under benign and in-principle achievable conditions, one can conceptualize a world that does not continuously rely on the collective management of force. The nature-based web of interactions that follow on play has no outer limit to separate it from a supposedly harsh public arena.

These characters of the object relations worldview are muted and limited in Fairbairn, who views the sovereign state, along with its coercive facet, as an indispensable level of organization precisely because it is separate from the private logic of attachment and emotional engagement: only by becoming a civic, political actor in an environment that pays him or her no particular attention, may the individual manifest the level of integration which is the essence of psychic health. But in the object relations tradition taken as a whole, this perception is not dominant. Rather than being ignored, Fairbairn's concepts of the child as primarily object-seeking and of integration as the ability to engage with others are recruited into a worldview which does not follow Fairbairn's notion of politics. From Ian Suttie's first, explicit effort to refute Freud's entire worldview to Winnicott's vision of play as expanding into culture, the notion of a dynamic private sphere that ultimately diminishes the role of policing, governments and formal institutions was the one favoured by the analysts. A healthily stable, trusting and communicative personality is not preoccupied with existential danger, and the society based on such personalities does not emphasize the need for the collective use of force. Accordingly, that society does not prioritize those organs where the collective use of force is debated and decided. The providing state is an extension of the home, not only in the sense of safeguarding the conditions for the family in a way that is analogous to what the family does for the child, but also in the sense of replicating the home's patterns of enabling and empowering that are conducive to communication, play and creativity. The state and the activities that take place around it do not have to be thought of as a specialized realm partitioned from the rest of human life. The sphere they operate in can instead be gradually, if never perfectly, absorbed into the comprehensive and multilayered totality that is that life.

The social worldview implied by the object relations perspective interfaced with a broader intellectual environment characteristic of the midcentury. That environment enabled the implementation of liberal welfare-state policies, but it also contained other political standpoints, marking a rising consensus on what Atlantic democracy was. The interface between this consensus and object relations thought is apparent when Winnicott is compared to Popper. Credited with formulating the philosophical justification for all Western democracies, whatever their declared ideological premises, Popper based his vision of the tolerant, loosely federated open society on the ability to freely exchange and debate ideas. The motivations of the participants in this discussion, the relations between them and the dynamic of their conversation resemble those of transitional space and play in Winnicott's work. The participants seek response and are therefore prepared to risk dearly held certainties, thus creating a link between the contents of their own mind and the surrounding reality. The discussion on which the open society relies is an intermediate, intersubjective level between individual interior and objective exterior. The responses offered by the interlocutors change each participant's views, and accordingly create new possibilities that exceed the cognitions that each of the discussants has started with. These developments take place in transition and play as well, leading, in Winnicott's case, to a vision of a democratic culture in which the state's role becomes technical, as it does in Popper's open society. Intersubjective communication, Popper and Winnicott suggest separately, is the locus of creativity and therefore of liberty. It should be safeguarded by political institutions. For both authors, the expected long-term effects of the freedom granted to individuals within the protected, essentially private sphere where discussion and play take place include the transformation and diminishment of the civic arena along with its institutions.

If Popper shows the synchronic resonance of the ideology implied in object relations theory, then Benjamin shows its diachronic characters of durability and adaptability. Owing to its expressly programmatic, agenda-setting nature, Benjamin's work propels ideological potentialities that were partially submerged in the earlier authors closer to the surface. In particular, her theory manifests the synergy between an idealistic perception of parenting and motherhood on the one hand, and a tendency to thin out the distinctness of civic and political engagement, on the other hand. If the first bond can be configured to enable the growth of personalities who combine confident self-realization with benevolent sociability, then that bond has the potential to structure and inform the entire society. The ensuing civilization does not depend on enforcement, collective defence and the bodies where decisions on these matters are taken. The intersubjective potentiality of the relationship between mother and child is the basis of a pre-political, universal and natural society by the measure of which institutional and civic bodies should be assessed and critiqued. And as that first bond is structured by the universal, nature-based roles of parent and child, its reach exceeds the formal egalitarianism of the civic sphere, which is by comparison artificial and shallow. A top-down, holder-held, expert-client relationship is subtly placed as superior to the relationships of strictly identical legal personas.

The phrase 'from the cradle to the grave' was coined to describe the mission and the mandate of the mid-twentieth-century welfare state. It meant that government was responsible for the entire span of the citizen's life. But it can be interpreted more broadly, as denoting the comprehensive character of welfare-state liberalism as a worldview that aspires to cover the minutest units and most rudimentary experiences simultaneously with the furthest reaches of public life, neglecting no facet of human experience. Its advocates often referred to ideas about the family and early life as their legitimizing basis, using that basis to formulate a justification for government to deal with wide, previously private aspects of its constituent individuals' lives, starting from birth and ending at no particular point. In object relations theory, the importance of the cradle was further elaborated and stressed. When understood as a political argument, the theory also entails that the dynamics that mark the first relationship may, when correctly approached and secured by the surrounding society, expand to enfold civilization as a whole. The nursery becomes the paradigmatic, foundational site for that civilization. Its rationale does not encounter a limit beyond which a different, political one replaces the rationale of the first bond. While featuring as a prominent theory of mind in an unprecedentedly prosperous and free society whose public institutions are informed by historical models of liberal democracy, object relations theory departs from historical liberalism's separation of the civic and political realm from the private one. This character, in this particular psychology, accords with a wider twentieth-century trend, in which liberal democracy is increasingly equated with a horizon where the multiplex, essentially voluntary and thus private sites secured by the constitutional state are expected to gradually diminish that state's significance, along with the significance of the various activities entailed by efforts to shape the state.

Unless liberals, and other adherents of the constitutional and democratic perspective initially believed in the distinctness of the political sphere and in the autonomy of politics, it is difficult to see how the idea of democracy itself could be sustained. If we accepted that a fundamental form of knowledge that determines right and wrong applied in the same way to all our activities, we would place ourselves at the discretion of experts who specialize in that knowledge while we could become freer to engage with other pursuits. No final decision by an egalitarian electorate would be needed, and the frustrations of public life as we know it would be obviated. But regardless of such considerations, twentieth-century liberals appear to gradually diminish the autonomy of politics. As a specialized discipline with a say on what constitutes the entire span of human life, object relations psychoanalysis is in some ways complicit in that process, as it reads the dynamics of the cradle and the nursery into everything else. The bouts of gender-based and ethnic supremacism that appear in some object relations tracts are therefore not wholly incidental. The elitism they harbour points to a profounder tendency towards a managerial perspective that blurs the distinction between politics, on the one hand, and scientific, medical and clinical knowledge, on the other hand. Such a perspective defines healthy and sick, good and bad, higher and lower, a tendency that can show as forms of ethnic and gender supremacism. Such elitism is the corollary to the theory's naturalist optimism and the priority it places on integration: ultimately, there are no issues that cannot be covered by the insights derived from the theory.

If one can agree to an extent with Benjamin's (2018: 28) assertion that we should not 'sunder the psychology of reciprocal recognition at the level of individual attachment from reciprocal recognition at the level of social rights', one should still be careful enough to concede that the applicability of that statement requires a limiting qualification. Beyond it, the issue can no longer be that of recognition or psychology. It becomes one of taking a collective existential decision on a question for the resolution of which nobody can provide us with ethical, scientific or clinical guidelines. Without such a boundary, the hierarchies of private life – parent and child, teacher and student, expert and client – invade the space where citizens should be equally empowered, and democracy ceases to be viable.

Reference

Benjamin, J. (2018). *Beyond doer and done to*. New York: Routledge.

Index

For Product Safety Concerns and Information please contact our EU
representative GPSR@taylorandfrancis.com
Taylor & Francis Verlag GmbH, Kaufingerstraße 24, 80331 München, Germany

www.ingramcontent.com/pod-product-compliance
Ingram Content Group UK Ltd.
Pitfield, Milton Keynes, MK11 3LW, UK
UKHW022355190926
475702UK00015B/2298
* 9 7 8 0 3 6 7 7 6 1 6 5 3 *